A Rainbow Book

HAIR
Surviving the Fall

Sara Romweber, Ph.D.

Rainbow Books, Inc.
FLORIDA

616.546
Rom

Library of Congress Cataloging-in-Publication Data

Romweber, Sara, 1937–
   Hair : surviving the fall / Sara Romweber.
      p. cm.
   Includes bibliographical references and index.
   ISBN 1-56825-093-2 (trade softcover : alk. paper)
   1. Baldness—Psychological aspects. I. Title.
   RL155.R66 2004
   616.5'46—dc22

                                                2004003836

Published by Rainbow Books, Inc., P. O. Box 430,
Highland City, FL 33846-0430

Editorial Offices and Wholesale/Distributor Orders
Telephone: (863) 648-4420 • Email: RBIbooks@aol.com

Individuals' Orders
Toll-free Telephone (800) 431-1579 • http://www.AllBookStores.com

Permissions
TIZIANO: Maria Maddalena — Galleria Palatina — Firenze, with the
permission of the Italian Ministry of Fine Arts and Cultural Works,
reproduction or duplication prohibited.
Sara Romweber's photo by Sue Ann Miller.
Cover art from the Joyce Buckner Collection.

First edition 2004
10 09 08 07 06 05 04   5 4 3 2 1
Printed in the United States of America

To all of the individuals
who spoke with me at length about
the emotional experience of
losing their hair.

Without your willingness to
come forth and share your feelings
this book would not have
been possible.

Contents

ACKNOWLEDGMENTS

I've often read an author's "acknowledgments" with interest —
and at the same time wondered how so many people could become
involved in the writing and publication of a single book. Now I know.

Special thanks go to Dr. Marcia Salner and to my fellow students at Saybrook Graduate School and Research Center who were
present at the inception of my doctoral research project, and who
later encouraged me to write this book. You know who you are.

Thanks to Laura Poole for her excellent editing, her useful suggestions, her sensitivity — and, above all, for her positive, pleasant,
and fun-loving spirit. You are great to work with, Laura.

Heartfelt thanks go to my two good friends and colleagues, Dr.
Ann Freeman and Dr. Meggan Moorhead, who followed my research
with interest and later offered positive encouragement, excellent advice, and abiding support during the writing of this book.

A sincere thank you goes to Allessandra Bertini for her diligent
assistance in helping me secure permission from the *Soprintendenzo
speciale per il Polo Museale fiorentino* in Florence, Italy, to use a
picture of a painting of Mary Magdalene (Titian), housed in the Galleria Palatina (in Florence). Her help was invaluable. Love and gratitude also go to my good friends, Drs. Ed and Hélène Montgomery,
for their help in translating letters faxed to me from the museum
officials, and above all for their generous spirits and warm support.

I especially want to thank my younger sister and brother-in-law,
Sheila and Larry Morin, who offered constant encouragement —
and devoted time, energy, and creative thought in search of a title.
And to Cris, who — having lost her hair during chemotherapy —
made excellent title suggestions.

My love and special thanks go to all the other members of my
family: my mother (Mary Jo Hammond), my brother (Henry), and
my older sister (Linda Franklin) for their brave endurance through

all of my giant endeavors. And to my children: Paul, Steven, Joe, Luke, Sara, Monica, and "Dex," who gave me the time and space to write — each helping in his or her own special way. Thanks go to Paul for his ongoing interest in the project (and special thanks just for *being proud of me*). Thanks go to Steven, who — early on — assured me over and over again that the subject matter was important and *timely*. To Joe and his lovely wife, Jackie, a special thank you for their encouragement, and for their enthusiastic support. Heartfelt thanks go to Luke (also a writer) for his excellent and appropriate suggestions, and for his constant interest and support. I am much obliged to Roger Sanders for his thoughtful guidance and ongoing support — and most of all for his being a loyal friend. A debt of gratitude goes to my daughter, Sara, for quietly tolerating my computer illiteracy — and most of all, for allowing me to tell the story of her (at the age of five) being led unknowingly to the hair salon by a female relative. A deep and loving thank you goes to Monica for keeping me well supplied in office materials, and for offering constant, positive support. Finally, a warm thank you to Dexter for his kind and sweet way of being in the world, and just for being Dexter. (And special thanks to all of you for helping me select the most appropriate "author's photograph.")

Grateful thanks go to Betty Wright and to the entire staff at Rainbow Books, Inc. You have to be the most reasonable, patient, and fun people in the world. You made this easy!

I finally want to thank my clients — especially B.T., K.J., D.K., A.S., and L.V. — who knew that this book was being published. Almost all of you said, "That's awesome." For those wonderfully spirited words, I am pleased.

Sara (Sally) Romweber

THE MANE COURSE

The Crowning Blow

My mother tells a story about herself that must have happened sometime in the 1920s. She was about nine or ten years old, and she

> Throughout history, hair has been considered not just ornamental but magical.
> — Diane Ackerman

had come down with typhoid fever during an epidemic of that terrible disease. She was quite seriously ill because the family was quarantined. "They roped off the block," she said, "to keep people away from the house." My mother's illness began during the hot summer months and lingered into the fall, so she was absent from school when classes resumed in September.

"My hair fell out," she says. This is the part that she talks about. She remembers every detail — being afraid that it wouldn't grow back in, her mother scanning her head with a bright light. Believing that it would grow back faster, my grandmother took my mother to a barber and asked that he clip the few remaining straggly hairs close to the scalp. "When he swung the chair around for me to look in the mirror," she said, "I shrieked! I was so upset. And so was Mama. I can see her face yet in pity for me." My mother's hair grew back, of course, but not before she was well enough to return to school.

She speaks intimately about the day she returned to her classroom. One of the rules of her small elementary school was that children were not allowed to wear hats while indoors. She was spared humiliation, however, by a kind and compassionate teacher who broke the rule and allowed her to keep her head covered with a little hat, "a Madge Evans, dark blue straw, with a brim that turned up all the way around, trimmed with a blue program ribbon." The teacher told the children that my mother had been very ill, and made a soft but direct announcement that "Mary Jo will be wearing a hat to school for an unspecified length of time."

I have listened to this story all my life. I have imagined my mother during those long, hot summer days, lying in bed with a raging fever, sometimes in delirium. I have imagined her returning to school, sitting at her small desk wearing her little straw hat, trying to act as if nothing were wrong. I've thought to myself, "How mortifying! Especially for a young girl." Even as a small child I was far more affected by my mother's story about her hair loss than the fact that she had had a terrible illness and might have died, as many did.

THERE'S NO DOUBT ABOUT IT

Hair is very important to humans. We love it, hate it, become angry with it, dutifully care for it — and we mourn if there is a loss. Close friends and family members mourn with us. It's a high-maintenance relationship that, if all goes well, is lifelong. There's no doubt about it: Our hair matters to us. It's a little like having a lover. When it's acting and responding in a way that we like, we feel comfortable and secure. When it isn't — commonly known as a bad hair day — we feel uneasy and out of sorts.

Women fuss over their hair in a multitude of ways; men can have the same kind of devotion. Male rock stars let their hair grow long. Some men hide the gray in their hair. Nowadays, men seek hair stylists instead of barbers. Cancer patients have occasionally been known to refuse radiation and chemotherapy treatments for fear of losing their hair — and those who do opt for this treatment frequently say that losing their hair was the worst part of their cancer experience.[1] Many men fret and worry about hair loss, and women who lose their hair grieve deeply. Many attempt to hide this unwanted change and closely guard their secret.

There are several theories about why hair matters so much to humans, and they all suggest that this part of the body has an important and meaningful history. Social anthropologists say that hair has been essential to the human species in matters of courtship and mating, indicating that it has served a purpose far beyond simply adorning the head or enhancing one's appearance. The speculation here is that in the early days of human evolution, males who had long and glorious hair — which made them look huge and fierce — successfully frightened off their competition for mates. In addition, women with long, healthy hair were more likely to be chosen as wives. Consequently, our hairiest ancestors survived through their conquest (and submission) and parented the next generation.[2]

Other folks, particularly zoologists, believe that the hair serves as a protective hood, saying that it shields the head (and brain) from the direct gaze of the sun.[3] The hair on the head may also provide a buffer or cushion for the skull and brain. Much like the eyelashes and brows protect the eyes and the tiny hairs inside the ears and nostrils prevent the entry of insects and dust, the scalp hair may act as a barrier against a blow to the head.[4]

Others say that hair is simply a social accessory; people can be creative about hairstyles — and those creations reveal something about the individual. One of my male clients said, "I can look at a woman, I can look at her hair, and tell something about her personality. You know, bossy ... mean ... sweet." Hairstyles can and do make statements about who we are. A particular style may reveal something about one's tendency to be outgoing or shy or may indicate an association with a certain group. It goes without saying that hair is the ultimate gender sign.[5] Moreover, hairstyles reflect something about current attitudes — especially attitudes about sex, sin, and society.[6]

The scalp hair is a fundamental, immensely durable part of one's physical being, continually growing out of, and for the most part, remaining attached to the head, with one poignant twist: The hair survives one's death. At no time has this fact been more evident or touched human spirits more deeply than when the content committee for the United States Holocaust Memorial Museum of Auschwitz-Birkenau received a box containing approximately twenty pounds of human hair among a shipment of artifacts. Members of the committee, particularly family members of Holocaust victims, viewed the curls, braids, and long locks of women's hair differently than the mirrors, razors, toothbrushes, and other personal belongings. One committee member expressed the fear that her own mother's hair might be in the pile of braids and locks, and announced that she did not want her mother's hair on display.[7] This abundance of hair — intended to symbolize torture and death — may actually have seemed more like an eerie symbol of everlasting life. Perhaps in viewing these tactile remains, there was an uncomfortable feeling among the committee members that the spirits of the victims were present along with their hair. The horror of the Holocaust was suddenly comprehensible in a much more personal way.

Hair is sexual, psychoanalysts say. But the sexual significance of hair is believed to be buried in the subconscious mind — a result of living in a progressively more civilized world. The suggestion here is that people use head hair for sexual expression subconsciously because it is a convenient and acceptable substitute in a world that struggles with its rules about sexuality (like who can have sex, when they can do it, who they can do it with).[8]

The idea of hair being a sexual part of the body is also evident in certain religious and cultural practices. For centuries, the hair of women in religious orders was required to be completely covered. From my own years in a Catholic girls' boarding school, I remember that if just one strand of hair wiggled out from a sister's headdress, she would quickly return to her private quarters and force the wayward lock back into confinement. Because the sight of a woman's hair was believed to evoke sexual feelings, Catholic women old and young for years had to wear a hat, a scarf, or some type of head covering when entering church.[9]

The symbolism of the hair on the head is ancient and complex. Those who have studied ritual behavior say that it frequently represents a kind of spiritual energy, indicating that it has a godlike quality. In these situations, the hair appears to be a metaphorical expression or symbol of the life force. This is easy to understand when we remember that for most of us the hair experience is a constant process (or cycle) of growth, change, separation, and sometimes loss — much like life.[10] In some societies it goes beyond symbolism. For example, there is a strong belief in many cultures that a connection actually exists between the hair and the soul. "North American Indians thought that the hair imprisoned the soul," said Wendy Cooper, "and that by scalping an enemy they captured the soul and prevented it from escaping and returning to seek its revenge."[11]

Whether we understand it or not, a sexual association with the scalp hair appears to be strong for both genders. Most of us know that playing with one's hair can be a flirtatious gesture, such as when one curls a strand around one's finger. Those of us who are old enough to remember will never forget Veronica Lake's sexy blond hair draped ever so slightly over one eye, and Bette Davis tossing her head to flip the bangs out of her face. Today's famous sexy hair would probably belong to Farrah Fawcett and Goldie Hawn.

Whatever the reasons are for having hair, one cannot argue that it is an important and integral part of the physical body, intimately connected with one's entire being. Hair is "as much part of us as our skin," wrote Cooper, "firmly linked to our blood supply." It reflects the general state of health of one's body (as does skin),[12] and can also reflect the state of one's emotional health (as stress has frequently been identified as a cause of hair loss).

So, why do we feel the way we do about our hair? Why is losing one's hair such an emotional experience? I openly proposed this question several years ago when discussing topics for dissertation research, and I was immediately encouraged by friends, family, fellow students, and faculty to find the answer. I decided that individuals who had actually lost their hair could best provide the answers.

I spoke at length with men and women who were experiencing hair loss, and they did provide answers to my questions. Their voices — along with historical, psychological, and cultural information — help us understand the emotional experience of hair loss.

MY MANE SOURCES

There were twenty primary sources of my research. Ten Caucasian males, six Caucasian females, and four African American females. Only two were completely bald — both of them women. Several others had experienced total hair loss, but it had been temporary. Most were experiencing partial baldness, which appeared to be a continuing process of losing hair. All of them had sought medical treatment in hopes of growing their hair back. Their ages ranged from 21 to 48. They had various occupations, everything from health care providers to computer programmers. Some were college students, several were in graduate school. A few were unemployed.

Brief profiles of these study subjects are presented here. Their words and feelings are described throughout the book. To protect confidentiality, all of their names have been changed.

—The Men—

Don was 29 years old and single when I met him. He was a college student trying to complete a four-year degree with plans to enter law school. Don had no hair on the top of his head, and he had let the hair on the sides and back grow about two inches long. He said that he had been losing his hair since he was 17 and that it was due to male pattern baldness. He was candid, congenial, and humorous. He dressed casually, and he appeared to be fairly spontaneous in all aspects of his life.

Walt was 26 years old and married. He, too, was experiencing male pattern baldness. When he talked about his hair, he said, "It's getting thin all over. Mostly, it's just my hairline is going back and back and back." He said that he noticed that his hair was receding when he was about 20 years old. He had an old picture of himself that showed the amount of hair he used to have. He looked like Troy Donahue (Dorothy McGuire's son in *A Summer Place*) back then. He said that he had resolved most of the painful feelings about his hair loss and that it had been a difficult process. He said that he wanted to share his feelings about the experience.

Bret was 35 years old and married. He said that he had been dealing with male pattern baldness since his early 20s. His hair loss was noticeable in that he had a visibly receding hairline. But so far, he said, there had been no loss of hair on the top of his head. Losing his hair was a bigger problem for him emotionally during the years that he was single and dating. He did consider himself less attractive, but said that it wasn't as big a problem now that he was married and had children.

Jake was 27 years old. He had completed four years of college. He was working for a software company and taking a few graduate courses in computer science. He was a single guy, and he said that he had been experiencing male pattern baldness since he was 18. His hairline was visibly receding, and the hair on top of his head appeared to be thinning as well. He looked older than his stated age. Jake's body language matched the feelings that he shared about his hair loss. He said that he felt diminished.

Bruce was 25 years old. He said that he was married but was soon going to be separated. Bruce said that he had been dealing with male pattern baldness since the age of 20. He had a significantly receding hairline, but a normal amount of hair on the top and sides of his head. He said that he had been a competitive swimmer while in college, and that when he was a sophomore the swimmers shaved their bodies (including their heads) for a national swim meet; about a month later, when everyone else's hair was growing back in, his hair was growing very slowly. That was when he realized that he was going bald. He said that up until that time he had a head of thick, blond hair; losing it was causing him to feel depressed and concerned about attracting women.

Mark was 21 years old and single. He said that he realized that he was losing his hair when he was a junior in high school, and everyone teased him about it. He said that he really began to notice it in college, especially when he saw old pictures of himself from high school. He wore a baseball cap to our meeting, and when he removed it briefly, I noticed a visibly receding hairline, along with thinning hair across the top and sides of his head. He said that his father was bald, along with both of his grandfathers. He said that he had expected to lose his hair at some time in his life, but that it had been very distressing to lose it at such a young age. At that time, Mark was a senior in college.

Dave was 24 years old. He, too, was a senior in college and single. He said that he had been experiencing male pattern baldness since his freshman year. Like Don, he had a more extensive, horseshoe pattern of hair loss. The difference was that the remaining hair on the sides and back of his head was clipped short. He said that his freshman year in college was a stressful time for him and that losing his hair "didn't help things a bit." During our meeting, Dave was rather cavalier about his hair loss. He insisted that it didn't bother him much, and that he just wanted to share his experience. He did add that he was always relieved to find out that potential girlfriends had balding fathers . . . "I'm in!"

Ralph was a 37-year-old, married man. He worked in telemarketing. He said that he began losing his hair when he was 15 or 16 years old and that it was due to male pattern baldness. He said that he used to have a really nice head of hair; now he wore a cap (or hat) most of the time. He said that he felt great when he had a full head of hair, but now he didn't feel "complete." He said that he was worried about his self-image and how he looked to other people. He wore a baseball cap to our meeting.

Thomas was 48 years old and divorced. He said that he began losing his hair when he was about 25 years old. Thomas said that one concern about losing his hair was that he missed the protection, both from the sun and from the cold weather. He said that his hair used to provide warmth during the winter months and that he had experienced several severe sunburns on the top of his head. He said that he used to have really long hair during the 1970s, and that not long after that he began to lose it. He, too, was experiencing male pattern baldness. He said that he didn't feel that he was as attractive to women as he would be if he had hair.

Roger was 29 years old. He was single, and he said that he had been experiencing male pattern baldness since he was 18. When I met him he had a significantly receding hairline, but this didn't make him look particularly older. The remaining hair on the top and sides of his head was thick, dark, and healthy in appearance. He said that early on — when he first noticed that he was losing his hair — he was successful in getting it to grow back with a prescribed medical product. He said, "I was so excited! . . . I was back in high school again . . . I was extremely happy." Sadly, however, Roger had to stop using the product. He willingly (and nostalgically) talked about how his life had been different during the short time that he had a regrowth of hair. When I met Roger, he was once again experiencing hair loss.

—The Women—

Yolanda was a 37-year-old woman. She was divorced and had four children. She said that she was diagnosed with alopecia areata in 1991; over a period of four to five months she lost all of her scalp hair. (Alopecia areata is a term that simply denotes hair loss. It is a common condition, but the actual cause remains unknown.) Yolanda had worn a wig until approximately six months before I met her. At that time her hair was in the process of growing back in, and she was going without her wig much of the time. The new growth of hair was sparse and thin, but she styled it well. She was a very attractive woman, but she said that she hadn't felt secure around men until recently (when her hair began to grow back). When I met Yolanda, she was beginning to date. She was a spirited individual, and she shared her feelings about her hair loss eloquently.

Grace was 45 years old when I met her. She was married and had several small children. Grace said that she had experienced temporary hair loss in 1991, six months after she had been seriously ill. During the illness she endured a prolonged fever — somewhere around 105 degrees — which damaged the hair follicles and caused significant (but temporary) loss of her scalp hair. On the day of our meeting, she was wearing her hair down about her shoulders and it fell in a natural style about her face. She said that it was now like it had been before her illness. Her life had returned to normal.

Selena was 26 years old and recently married. She said that she began losing a significant amount of hair about eight months prior to our meeting. She said that it started with one small area, and then large sections began to fall out. She said that when she shampooed her hair, massive amounts came out; eventually the balding area was like a head band all around her head. When we met it was believed that her hair loss was due to using a specific type of birth control. However, she has recently learned that it was caused by a hair product she was using. Her hair is now growing back in.

Melissa was 25. She was single and had experienced alopecia areata and periods of total scalp hair loss since she was a small child. She said that her hair first fell out when she was four or five years old, grew back while she was in elementary school, and began falling out again when she was in high school. She said that when she was in her first year of college it all fell out for the last time. When I met her she was wearing a wig. She said that she only takes the wig off when she is at home, the doors are locked, and the shades are down. She doesn't have a boyfriend, and she does not date. She works as a health care technician in a nursing home.

Roberta was 36 years old. She was married and had several children. She was a stay-at-home mom. She said that about four years earlier she began to experience episodes of significant hair loss, and the doctors had been unable to give her an accurate diagnosis, mainly because several potential causes had been identified. Stress, along with a prescribed medication, however, were believed to have been the cause. She said that even though her hair grew back in, it had been a horrifying experience, and that she was noticing that it was happening again. She said that she couldn't bear to look in the mirror; she couldn't bear to see so much of her scalp through the strands of hair.

When I met **Angela** she was 34 years old and single. She is a well-educated and intelligent individual with a mental illness. She said that she had been diagnosed with bipolar disorder (manic-depressive illness), and she appeared to understand what that meant. She said that her first experience with significant hair loss was in 1991, two months after a serious suicide attempt (an overdose). She said that she was on the intensive care unit for six weeks and had not been expected to live. After she got home, her hair fell out. The doctors told her that the overdose was so severe that it had killed the hair follicles that were in that particular stage of growth (much like Grace's experience). At the time of our meeting, she was dealing with a second bout of major hair loss that had started about six months before. She said that this time it was related to stress. The day that I met with Angela, she was wearing a small kerchief to cover the balding areas.

Sheila was 32 year old, and at the time of our meeting she was single. She said that she was diagnosed with alopecia universalis when she was a small child. This is a form of alopecia areata in which there is a total absence of body hair (no eyebrows, lashes, etc.). When she was three years old Sheila's hair began to fall out in patches; she woke up one morning and found one of her little plaits on her pillow, and the next morning, another. She said that by the time she was four years old she was almost completely bald. Sheila wears a wig. She is an extremely attractive woman. Her makeup is flawless, and one would never know that her hair is not her own. When we met she was working as a bank teller.

Hattie was 44 years old when I met her. At the time of our meeting she was married and had teenaged children. She was experiencing a mild form of alopecia areata. She said that for ten years she had been under medical treatment trying to get her hair to grow back onto the balding areas of her scalp. She was receiving steroid injections directly into these areas — a treatment that supposedly stimulates the regrowth of hair. She said that she continually deals with bald spots and she generally lives without a fourth of her scalp hair. She appeared to be diligent about her treatments.

Joy was a 37-year-old woman with short, carefully styled hair. She was married and had a teenage daughter when we met. On that day, in the privacy of my office, she lifted her hair on the right side of her head and exposed a large, bald spot. She said that the hair in this area fell out approximately 15 years ago after her daughter was born, and it never grew back. She said that her doctor attributed the hair loss to her pulling her hair back tightly (into a bun or ponytail) over a long period of time. She said that she was never given a diagnosis but was told that this sometimes happens to African American females. She said that the hair in this area continued to fall out over a period of two years until it was just a large bald spot. She said that it had been a devastating experience — that she was self-conscious about it then, that she is self-conscious about it now.

Helen was a 38-year-old, white single female who had been experiencing female pattern balding since the age of 13. She said that the condition follows a more diffuse pattern of hair loss for women, rather than the receding hairline or crown hair loss that is typical for men. When I met Helen her hair was thinning all over her head. It was not quite shoulder length and was combed in a natural style about her face. I could easily see her scalp through the strands of hair. She said that unlike most female pattern baldness, her hairline was receding. She pulled her hair back and exposed a larger-than-normal forehead. She said that she wasn't shocked about her hair loss because hereditary baldness was "pretty much dominant in both males and females" on both sides of her family. She said that she had experienced a variety of painful emotions over losing her hair, but she was now in the process of trying to accept it. She said that she was always on the lookout for women who were balding to use as role models, but she frequently watches television shows that address cures for male pattern baldness in hopes of finding a reasonable solution for herself.

↭

People generally have highly emotional and personal feelings about hair — their own hair and sometimes other peoples' hair, especially the shorn remains of a loved one. Interestingly enough, the scalp hair appears to have no use or purpose in life whatsoever. A haircut that is too short — even hair loss — is neither life-threatening nor restricting of one's ability to function. So, how can we feel so strongly about a part of the body that seems to have no use?

It may appear to be all wrapped up in vanity and romance, but in so many ways the hair is an important and symbolic part of the human body. It characterizes our personality, our personal identity, and our sexuality. Hence, its loss — for both men and women — is likely to have painful, emotional consequences. According to the literature and to the people that I spoke with, head hair does indeed have a purpose and a function.

Part I

UNDERSTANDING THE IMPORTANCE OF HAIR

CHAPTER ONE

THE SPREAD OF THE PEACOCK'S TAIL

The Biological Purpose of Head Hair

RECEDING, REACTING, AND RETREATING

Don walked into my office and took the lid off of the candy jar. He said that he was hungry and asked if he could have some. He then proceeded to finish every piece. He was comfortable with himself, he seemed to feel comfortable with me, and he was there to tell me what was on his mind. In getting acquainted he said that he was a college student, in pre-law, and was working as a bartender to make ends meet.

> *We can picture our remote ancestor as he stands defiant on his hind legs, a mane of shaggy hair reaching to his shoulders, with beard bristling and glaring eyes accentuated by the arched eyebrows above and curling moustaches below, and with bare cheeks and forehead flushed in anger.*
>
> — Dr. C. B. Goodhart

Don said that prior to entering college he had lived in a predominantly all-male environment; he had attended an all-male prep school — where he was voted "Most Likely to Recede" — and most of his family members were male. He said that he hadn't had much experience socializing with females before entering a coed university, and his concerns about his appearance (his baldness) had made this transition difficult.

Don described his hair loss as a "horseshoe," meaning that he had no hair on the top of his head, and the hair on the sides and back of his head was thick and longer. He stated repeatedly that he was distressed about losing his hair and that he was simply trying to make the best of it. It seemed that most of his concerns were about attracting women and simply not feeling comfortable with his appearance. He said:

> As for a guy . . . it's like, every sexy man I see has hair. And I think, God! I must not even be in the game here. It goes back to this kind of neurotic thing again, where you're out with your girlfriend and she may be looking at some guy. And then the way the neurosis kicks in, is that you think . . . okay, the guy catches her eye and he thinks, "Oh, she's with somebody who's bald. Maybe I have a chance." You know, maybe that gives him more of an impetus to try to create a problem for me. Yeah, I've done a lot of thinking about this. It's been a big deal.

More than anything, Don seemed to feel that any man with a full head of hair could easily come between him and his girl. He said, "I'm not a fighter, and I'd just rather not be in that situation, period, for any reason. And, being bald just might be one more reason why that might happen." He stated repeatedly during our meeting, "I'm kinda out of that loop."

How important is hair when it comes to dating and mating? It is important now, and according to many anthropologists, it was quite important to our hairy ancestors.

In the Cave

If we believe in the evolutionary process described by Darwin (1936) — that the human species survived through the principle of natural selection (or survival of the fittest) — then our ancestors were originally a species covered with a thick growth of bodily hair.[1] This covering served many purposes for early humans. It kept them warm, protected them from scrapes and abrasions, and offered a handhold for the young. Additionally, it might have provided a little camouflage in their dangerous surroundings.[2]

It is impossible to know how this natural covering of hair disappeared. One theory is that as the earth's climate began to warm up, the furry coats were shed for comfort. Another theory is that the discovery of fire and the use of animal skins for bodily protection reduced the need for a thick coat of fur. Shedding the bodily hair might also have helped the primates move more quickly through the forests when chasing prey or escaping danger. A naked body would also allow for greater mobility in the water once the hunting apes moved from the forest to the shore in search of food.[3]

It has even been speculated that losing the bodily hair allowed for closer physical comfort (or intimate contact) between mating couples and that bare skin heightened tactile sensation, adding to sexual pleasure and physical awareness.[4] This is all guesswork, of course. No one can ever be certain about the reasons why we lost most of our bodily hair, leaving us with only a few patches of coarse growth.

The most believable reason for our ancestors having shed most of their hair, however, is that when they began hunting in hot, tropical areas, they evolved into a species that could survive the heat. The human body has a wide distribution of sweat glands through which heat is generated, and bare skin adds to the efficiency of its cooling system. Little or no metabolic heat is produced in the brain and scalp, so there would be no advantage in not having hair on this part of the body.[5] Because the cranial hair protects the head from the glare of the sun, it would allow the tropical mammals to be more comfortable while hunting in the daylight hours.[6]

Nonetheless, it is believed that the cranial hair has remained a part of the human body for more than just mechanical reasons. Experts agree that the patches of hair that remain have something to do with sexual significance.[7] Darwin was the first to make this suggestion. He said the most probable reason for our retaining a few patches of bodily hair served "ornamental purposes," part of the "sexual selection" process (one sex being modified in relation to the other sex).[8]

> This form of selection depends, not on a struggle for existence in relation to other organic beings or to external conditions, but on a struggle between the individuals of one sex, generally the males, for the possession of the other sex. The

result is not death to the unsuccessful competitor, but few or no offspring.[9]

Within a furry species, the female didn't choose a mate with the most impressive hair (although Darwin thought this was the case). Actually, our ancestors' mating ritual went something like this: The male with the most impressive hair — or he who could make it look that way — frightened away his rivals, got his girl, and fathered the next generation. Hence, the head hair played a major role in obtaining a partner and successfully producing offspring.

The idea of hair growth being part of the "sexual selection" process makes sense when we remember that much of the patchiness of human hair grows during puberty and cannot possibly be associated with a need for warm fur. Along with drawing attention to the sexual organs, some patches of hair (under the arms and on the crotch) hold sexually stimulating aromas — important odors that are exciting and pleasing to many people.[10] Furthermore, if the patches of hair that remain were intended as protective devices, women and children would have more hair than they do. After all, they are generally smaller and more fragile than males.[11]

One zoologist in particular noted that certain species of monkeys have patches of hair on their heads very similar to humans; it develops during puberty, is found only among the males, and is used during intermale rivalry. In evolutionist language this is called *epigamic* hair, which means that it is a sign of sexual dominance.[12] The lion's mane is an example of epigamic hair, as it is used as a scare technique during sexual fighting. Another example is the decorative nature of Native Americans when dressed for battle. Historically, they adorned themselves with plumes and feathers in order to create a more impressive, frightening appearance when on the warpath.[13]

"It is an interesting and important observation," wrote C. B. Goodhart, "that, despite the loss of our body fur, some living races of mankind can still show as luxuriant a display of typical epigamic hair as any of the other primates."[14] It is also an interesting and important observation that in the modern world of humans, hair continues to play a major role in mate selection (and intermale rivalry). Jake said that "as long as physical attributes are as dominant as they are in the world, and in picking sexual partners, [scalp hair] is going to be a wedge point between those who have and those who haven't."

Bret agreed. "Baldness equals some sort of inadequacy, or less desirability, or something like that." Don said that he thought there was an "instinctive competition to mate," and having hair was "something to give somebody a more competitive edge over somebody else."

Was She Dragged By Her Hair?

Hair competition, however, was not and is not exclusively a male sport. Goodhart suggests that our female ancestors could (and would) grow their hair long (sometimes below the waist) and that it was used to attract a mate.[15] This means that women were, perhaps, rejected or not fought over if they lacked a generous amount of heavy, shiny hair.

Almost all of the women that I spoke with implied (without realizing it) that these theorists were right. Angela said that she believed that hair had a lot to do with one's sexuality. "I think if there was a sexual competition between two women over one man — the man choosing between two women — I think the girl with the pretty golden locks is going to get chosen." In her opinion, hair is "a very primordial sort of thing . . . sick animals lose their hair, and if the head hair is abnormal, then I think this kind of sets off some kind of prehistoric alarm that says, "Don't mate with this animal, don't come in contact with this animal."

Roberta reported a long, intense, and passionate relationship with her hair. She seemed to know (instinctively) the significant role that it plays in finding a partner.

> As you grow up and become interested in finding a relationship, then you realize that your appearance is part of that attraction. Men can be bald and sexy, but hair is an accepted part of a female's appearance. It's part of a female's allure. I mean, hair is part of one's attempt to find a mate.

A woman's head of hair is not so different (if at all) from a man's head of hair. Why then does it receive so much more attention in the area of mating? Cooper thinks that it has something to do with a woman's body being almost void of visible hair on her face and body, such that, "by contrast, her remaining largest area of hair has gained in desirability. By displacement a woman's head hair is to the male a symbol of her pubic hair and hence of her very womanhood."[16]

Women who have lost their hair seem to know that they are missing this sexual sign. Yolanda spoke about her fears of rejection. She said that she and her husband were not living together during the initial phase of her hair loss, and when she realized that he wanted a divorce, she said to herself, "Who in the world is going to want a divorced woman with four children who is going bald?" She said, "I just remember crying . . . really . . . I couldn't take it. I thought, *God! . . . forget about having four children! Bald! Nobody wants a bald woman!*"

Helen said that she had a fear (related to her hair loss) that stemmed from fantasies of rejection.

> I've been a single person my whole life, and it didn't alter my feelings of fear of rejection and growing old alone, and all of those feelings that I don't think are terribly uncommon. It's really associated with that feeling that we have of, like . . . you know, my problem is my loneliness and my solitude and, you know . . . if only I had that luxuriant head full of hair, the men would never be able to leave me alone.

"Head hair, together with well-rounded buttocks and breasts, have always been attractive to men," wrote Bernard Campbell,[17] and women seem to know this. Grace, who was married, spoke of the sexual ramifications of her baldness: "My husband, I noticed, was very cool to me. There was less lovemaking. You know, that kind of activity. And my husband . . . I mean, he wanted my hair long. That was the other thing that I knew."

And Sheila, who doesn't let men get "too close," said that she's afraid once a man finds out that she doesn't have any hair "it might change things."

> A lot of times I felt like maybe that's why I don't have a boyfriend. Maybe that's why I'm not married. Maybe that's the reason. I do think not having hair has a lot to do with not having a relationship and everything. I really do. If I feel like they're getting too close, asking a lot of questions that I don't want to answer, I know I push them away.

Our female ancestors may have had little choice in mate selection, but most modern women believe that they do have some control in the game of love. "The erotic appeal of a woman's hair is a complex matter of texture, color, scent, and movement," said Wendy Cooper,[18] and a woman does have control over most of these elements. She can color her hair, and perfume it, and she can move her head in such a way, setting her hair in motion, so that it will swing in a graceful, sexy manner. She can also play with a strand or two, always an inviting signal. It is simply part of the performance. Angela spoke about women who, when out in a crowd and looking for guys, start playing with a lock of their hair.

> It's just a way of showing that she can be touched. You know, we can't go to a bar and do this [she rubbed her breasts], saying, "Here, baby . . . this is what you can do with me." But she can . . . legally . . . in our society . . . she can play with her hair, and toss it back. You know, how many times have you seen that behavior . . . particularly among younger girls . . . girls who are nervous around boys . . . it's like mane-shaking among horses.

Yolanda said that, for her, "hair is part of the mating ritual."

> Head movement is very important. When you are losing your hair you lose a part of that . . . that ritual in mating . . . in sensuality. Hair is a part of womanhood. It's been a part of our ritual from the day we were born. Our mothers put bows in our hair . . . made our hair as attractive as possible. It was part of being a girl, of being a woman as you were growing up.

Angela and Yolanda are correct. Hair and head movement are a primal part of the mating ritual. According to Helen Fischer, women often nod or toss their heads in flirtation, setting their hair in motion. Animals, too, participate in the mating game with a tilt or toss of the head, while locked in a moment of anticipation.[19]

Hairiness on other parts of the female body — for example, a beard — is considered undesirable, of course. This, too, stems from our ancestors.[20] Goodhart wrote that a lack of hair on the female's face and chest evolved in response to our male ancestors "who liked their women with naked bodies as well as with a fine head of hair."[21] In no human race do maturing women normally have hair on their chest or face. And should hair appear in an unwanted place, they will actively seek to have it removed (even if it's a painful procedure). Most women seem to like their men hairy (symbolizing maturity and strength?[22]), but prefer their own bodies to be hair free (except for the head, of course).

It seems, then, that one of the key signs of masculinity or femininity has something to do with hair, especially where it is on the body and how much one has. The more hair displayed on a male (or female) body (i.e., arms, legs, chest, face) the more masculine he (or she) appears to be. [Of facial hair on our male ancestors, Darwin wrote, "Our male ape-like progenitors acquired their beards as an ornament to charm or excite the opposite . . ."[23]] Less body hair, on the other hand, is identified as a feminine trait, and is seemingly more desirable for females.

∽

The most probable reason for losing mass quantities of bodily hair during the course of evolution was probably to serve the process of sexual selection (one sex being modified in relation to the opposite sex). The hairier the male, the better his chances were of winning a battle (over a female) and mating. And females with long, healthy, luxurious hair were believed to be more desirable — thus chosen (or fought over) — as partners. Hence, good hair was seen as an asset (for both sexes) in partnering, perhaps indicating better health (more likely to reproduce) in a mate.

Thus, within the human species, hair has survived largely as an ornamental appendage and as a means of sexual attraction. Those who have a nice head of hair generally don't realize its powerful significance. In fact, they take it for granted. The full psychological and social importance of one's hair becomes shockingly clear, however, should a bald patch be found or one's hairline begins to recede. For a woman, loss of hair diminishes her sense of sexual appeal and perhaps lessens her chance of finding a mate; for a man, it fuels his fear of aging and impotence, badgering his self-confidence. Simply put, hair is a powerful sexual signal.

CHAPTER TWO

WAVELENGTHS

*The Public Importance of Hair and
the Private Effects of Its Loss*

A PUBLIC AFFAIR

I was a senior in high school,
my sixth and final year in a Catholic girls' boarding school. In that
closed environment I'm not sure
how I became aware of Gina
Lollobrigida and Sophia Loren
and their very sexy hair, but I remember thinking that they were

> Hair is perhaps our most powerful
> symbol of individual and group
> identity — powerful first because
> it is physical and therefore
> extremely personal, and second
> because, although personal, it is
> also public rather than private.
> — Anthony Synnott

gorgeous, voluptuous women, and I wanted to look like them. I was
16 years old, developing nicely, on the verge of liberation, and focusing more attention on my hair.

Notices were being placed everywhere that a photographer was
coming to take pictures for the school yearbook — a not-so-subtle
message that on that day we should look our best (i.e., pressed uniforms, starched collars). Hundreds of candid pictures were taken of
small groups of students participating in school activities: volleyball, class projects, religious services. And I was happily in the midst
of it all. I had restyled my hair, carefully defining little spit curls
around my face (much like my movie star idols) and hairsprayed
myself to perfection. I looked mature and sensual.

Several weeks later I heard my name called over the public address system. It was Sister Aileen asking me to come to the principal's office. Sister Aileen was a scary nun — the sour, harsh, punitive type, who rarely if ever smiled. She was waiting in the doorway of her office, and as I entered she handed me the proofs of all the photos I was in. All were quite flattering, and I was delighted. But she was furious! "You look like a loose woman! How could you do such a thing to your hair?" She rambled on and on, angry, heartless, and all-powerful. I sat stunned and humiliated. She called the photographer to come back and take all the pictures (of me) over. I glance through that musty, 1954 yearbook every now and then. I see pictures of a naive, innocent, and optimistic young girl. My hormones were squirming, but my hair was in place.

Hence, the ways we style our hair can send a message to the world about how we perceive ourselves at any given stage of life. It would be nice if this were our private and personal business, but the people around us get to know all about it — and generally, they take notice. Our hair is one of the few parts of the body that we can be freely artistic with; so closely related to the personality (or inner self), it's a way to express the self, especially the creative self. My sexy little wisps of hair told the nuns that I was becoming interested in boys (and in my own appearance). And to make matters worse, I was announcing it! The Catholic sisters did not want their girls to appear or be sensual. They Adamantly preached virgin-like qualities: purity, modesty, and reserve. They supported and encouraged motherhood, but not sex.

A particular hairstyle (or a change in hairstyle) can reflect a need to be true to oneself — whoever and whatever that self is at the time — plus a willingness to wear this badge of self-assurance. The story of women's hair has defined the process of women's liberation. As men have rebelled against a stuffy society's code of behavior, they, too, have changed the ways they wear their hair. Hair is a vital part of our public image — so much so that loss of it can be painful. Its value is priceless; its loss, devastating.

People experiencing hair loss generally don't talk about it; clearly, some individuals are just not bothered by it. But many are, and when they speak of their experience they reveal a surprising level of emotional distress. Both women and men speak of feeling insecure around the opposite sex (indicating a feeling of not measuring up to those who do have hair). Some say they feel self-conscious. Many individuals experiencing hair loss feel that their appearance simply does not convey to the public who they really are. Men are perceived (and treated) as older than their years, and women are viewed as asexual beings (a feeling also reported by men).[1] Jake, whose hair is receding, said he noticed right away that he was believed to be older than he was. He said that he wanted to be a young college kid, yet he knew that he was perceived as "near graduation, graduating, or something . . . you're young, and you have this young soul and everything. And all of a sudden your body around you is changing and making you be seen by others in ways that you don't consider yourself."

Roger, who began losing his hair right after high school, said that he lost his self-image (and sense of belonging) that summer. "You know, I wanted my classmates [in college] to see this kid who had grown up in this high school and had such a great time . . . and who he was. And what they were seeing was this guy with a receding hairline, who was very different than who they were."

We rely on our hair. It can make a powerful statement, a tool with which we speak without saying a word.

Historical Hairsay (Hers)

Nineteenth-century women didn't say much with their hair. It was an era that forbade a sensual appearance or overt sexual interest, and it was the woman's responsibility to keep this vigil. As Willett Cunnington wrote: "Those inaccessible charms were indeed exasperating; for who across an acre of crinoline could come to grips with such a subject? But it was the aim of the Perfect Lady to be ever slightly out of Man's reach."[2]

These women were a reserved, sympathetic, and romantic lot who were expected to cover nearly every inch of their bodies, including their hair. They wore large bonnets when out in public[3] — wide-brimmed head coverings tied gently beneath the chin — which successfully covered their hair, shielded their vision (and faces) from prospective suitors and kept them properly restricted so as not to disgrace themselves (or their families) with any improper or overt flirting with the opposite sex. Beneath each bonnet was an array of tight curls or braids (sometimes false) adorned with hair pins, flowers, combs, or bows.[4] The outside world, however, only saw the bonnets, as opposed to the women — obedient and submissive women who hid their hair as a symbol of modesty and restraint.

By the middle of the nineteenth century, bonnets disappeared. Hair (and faces) were becoming more visible, said Cunnington, as women began "to emerge from their seclusion and enter the world."[5] Discarding the bonnet was a relatively minor change, however, as throughout the remainder of the century women continued to bear lofty attitudes and keep their sexual distance, and their hairstyles said so. Written in a little bible for women on respectability, Charlotte Yonge said that when a woman reached a certain age, she was simply expected to put her hair up, to reduce it to "well-ordered obedience"[6] (perhaps like keeping one's legs crossed). Women were expected to have a sense of dignity about their hair. Unmanaged hair was simply "not consistent with the dainty niceness of true womanhood." Furthermore, said Yonge, "the loose unkempt locks of Sir Peter Lely's portraits" were not those of pure and dignified young women and matrons.[7] The carefully managed ways in which women arranged their hair made it perfectly clear that they were, indeed, still ever so slightly out of mens' reach. They had big hair (mostly false) and even bigger hats. Paul Poiret, a famous designer during the early 1900s, wrote, "I dined the other day in a fashionable restaurant. At the tables around me I noticed at least half a dozen women whose hair was dressed in exactly the same way, with the same number of puffs and switches."[8]

At the turn of the twentieth century women still had big hair (real and false), it was just under a smaller hat. This, too, would soon change. During World War I, the women who were helping out soon learned that less was better (and easier to manage). So they put away their puffs and switches and cut their hair. The bob announced a newfound freedom (and simplicity) for women.[9] The men were away, and women had to manage things. That was the beginning of the end of the hair police (and the sex police).

By the 1920s something else was going on: Women were being credited with sexual interest and sexual feelings. They began to dress more and more provocatively, and they dyed their hair blond — a bold statement of sexuality, for sure. Blonds were everywhere during and after this era, yet not all women were ready or eager to make so drastic a change. There was a stigma about being blond, something about being flighty or silly, and women were sometimes called dumb blondes — a label that may well have been unfair toward these whimsical, courageous, and daring young women. As Wendy Cooper reminds us, "the dumb blonde is often also the sexy blonde, whom gentlemen were once supposed to prefer."[10] It's quite possible that the blonde women of that era — especially the partying blondes known as flappers — were simply celebrating the end of a terrible war, having their men at home, and their recently acquired freedom.

Women must have made their first big leap into competing with men somewhere around this same time and saying so with their hair, because another, shorter hairstyle appeared during the 1920s: the Garçon (or, as known in England, the Eton Crop). This particular cut was a drastic and surprising change for women: cut short like a boy's and brushed straight back with the ears showing. It looked like a little cap on a small head — an effect that must have been elegant (and startling) and somewhat masculine.[11] According to J. Laver, many men did not like it:

> In vain old-fashioned gentlemen exclaimed that hair was a woman's crowning glory; in vain old-fashioned ladies strove to find a hat which they could possibly wear. There seemed to be no alternative; and it is an astonishing thought that in the years between 1925 and 1930 the vast majority of women in Western Europe, with the exception of Spain, must have cut off their hair.[12]

The 1930s were equally important for women's hair (and women's freedom), as women were, perhaps, relaxing their sexual guard a little more. The movies and their female stars were becoming popular, and hair — at least for the young, attractive glamour queens — was longer and flowing more naturally and sensuously. Many of the young women across the United States and Europe were successfully replicating this look at home, a subtle declaration that they were gaining an even greater sense of their sexuality and independence.[13] Older women, however, did not claim this right. The older gals stuck to the rules and kept their hair either short (sort of a Sophie Tucker look) or up, and often beneath a hat.

Another war captured our attention — World War II. Men went into combat, women went to work, and hair was kept simple. Some women wore a "done up on top, screwed into that ready-for-the-bath look," said Laver. Some wore a turban; many of the younger women simply let their hair hang loosely down around their shoulders.[14] Perhaps this loose, natural, sensible hair said something about the way women were beginning to view themselves: serious, focused, concerned, useful (yet feminine) human beings. Their hair said more about women's ability to make a contribution to the world and less about being tightly curled, jeweled, feathered decorations that hung on men's arms and pocketbooks.

After two world wars — after women had gone to work and tossed out their corsets, false hair pieces, long dresses, and bathing suits that concealed every curve — there were still women who arranged their hair in a stiffened and sprayed style, with their sexuality and freedom buried beneath it. (This was, coincidentally, during my boarding school days.) Maria Aldrich said that her mother's hair never blew in her face, never invited an embrace, was in effect, unapproachable. Maria also observed that along with becoming some man's wife (or some man's property), the hairstyles of these new brides changed noticeably and remained so for a very long time. Sculptured, molded, and carefully groomed, these hairdos were unnatural and unfriendly. "This was hair no one touched, crushed, or ran fingers through," said Aldrich. Somehow, in the presence of men, some women seemed to have difficulty simply letting their hair down.[15]

Nearly a decade later, when Jackie Kennedy's hairstyle was all the rage, many women still looked constructed, arranged, and sprayed (even Jackie herself). Their hair said, "I am untouchable, and I smell like hair spray." Were these lingering signs of an abstinence vigil? Possibly. Women were clearly being recognized as sexual beings and having sexual feelings. But until the women's movement, nice girls were not permitted to be too sensual or overly sexual (except in the movies), and their hair said so.

The 1960s arrived, along with the Pill. Women said quite a bit about this turn of events with their hair (as did men). Someone called it the decade of hair. Ways of arranging the hair were more natural and relaxed. There were even individuals who didn't bother with their hair at all: These folks were called hippies, and there was a fair number of women among them. "Hippies were immediately recognizable because of their rejection of accepted, conventional hair styles," wrote Cooper. "Their flowing, disheveled hair was in itself a badge of protest."[16] White women who were among this group of rebels in the 1960s and who longed to be like Joan Baez and Judy Collins wore their hair long and straight, a hairstyle that expressed contempt for the rigid thinking and stuffy ideals of their parents' generation.[17]

As the feminist movement blossomed in the 1970s — and a stand was being made toward equality (sexual and otherwise) — women who were ascending the ladder in the workplace began to cut their hair short once again. They may have felt that long hair was simply too feminine for the male-dominated business world. Moreover, short hair symbolized more masculine traits, such as logic and reason.[18] Again, short hair was also easier to manage, an important factor when there's a home, husband, and children to care for after a hard day at the office. But let's not overlook the fact that short hair on women (in business) might also be a covert way of saying, "My feelings are under control, I'll face you eye to eye, I won't flinch under pressure, you'll never see me cry."

There is yet another occasion when women seem to cut their hair short. It has something to do with motherhood, as many pregnant women (and new mothers) simply cut their hair off entirely. "It's easy to take care of," they say. Ackerman, however, suggests that this is a symbolic gesture. "A freshly bobbed new mother might be saying, in essence, 'I'm going to focus my life now on nurturing my family; I'm not available for flirtation."[19] Some new mothers cut their hair and don't know why, like Maria Aldrich's sister: "Once, after having her first baby, the dangerous time for women, she recklessly cut her hair to just below the ear. She immediately regretted the decision and began growing it back as she walked home from the salon, vowing not to repeat the mistake."[20]

A change in hairstyle can speak of many things for a woman, even a private transition, one that she herself isn't aware of yet (and if she were, she wouldn't tell just anyone). Even a dream of change in hair (i.e., color, style, length) can coincide with a change in one's life.[21] Aldrich wrote humorously and candidly about her mother's desire for life changes, projected through plans for a new and different hairstyle, spoken in "conspiratorial, almost confessional, tones."

With Julie [her hairdresser], my mother discussed momentous decisions concerning hair color, and the advancement of age and what could be done about it, hair length and its effects upon maturity, when to perm and when not to perm, the need to proceed with caution when a woman desperately wanted a major change in her life like dumping her husband or sending back her newborn baby and the change she could effect was a change in her hair.[22]

Carefully guarded feelings and personal transitions, however, are not always so private (especially among the rich and famous) and hair tells all. Soon after Diana, Princess of Wales, and her husband, Prince Charles, were separated, Diana appeared (on stage) in New York City wearing a straight, deep royal blue gown, with her hair cut shorter, seriously slicked back, and smoothed behind her ears. (She previously chose a short, relaxed look, with long, soft bangs.) When Monica Lewinsky was interviewed on the Barbara Walters Show (before Ken Starr had completed his investigation of President Clinton), gone was the loose, floppy, sexy, dark hair. Instead she bore shorter, smaller, neater, controlled hair, much like Princess Diana's new hair. Whether an intentional creation to impress the public, or a serious sign of newfound discipline, Monica's hair spoke of maturity, reserve, and refinement.

A woman's hair is so vital to her social and emotional existence that the very idea of hair loss is big news, especially for a well-known beauty. When Princess Caroline of Monaco suddenly lost all of her hair, the sight of her bald head created a tabloid stampede. Reports were that she looked more like a prisoner in a concentration camp than one of the world's most attractive women. Speculations about the cause were rampant. Her brother finally addressed the problem publicly and calmed everybody down with the news that Caroline's baldness was due to a skin problem and that her hair would grow back.[23]

Wigs, which have been available for centuries, have aided women in hiding their baldness and in keeping a carefully guarded secret. Regardless, it's a lonely world for women who experience significant hair loss — a secret world in which they often hold themselves apart from people who have hair. Both Melissa and Sheila have lived their lives (thus far) without hair, and each wears a wig. Melissa said, "I haven't told a lot of people. Most people that I've met don't know. They might realize that I wear a wig, but they don't know why." Sheila agreed:

Even with close friends . . . I have a lot of close friends and they don't know. They may suspect, and wonder if I've had cancer or something . . . but I've only told a few. I don't tell. It's nothing that I share. There's even some of my distant family members that know that my hair came out when I was little, but they don't know that the problem continued. They think that this is my hair. They never knew that it just didn't grow back.

Historical Hairsay (His)

Men competed with women for hair attention during earlier times, appearing in long hair, curls, braids, bows, and enormous powdered wigs, but this changed sometime during the beginning of the nineteenth century. Wigs began to disappear, and hair for men became more natural. "Hair was unpowdered," wrote Richard Corson. "It was considerably shorter, and eventually, facial hair was almost universally worn."[24] Shorter, simply arranged hair required less care and was less cumbersome for men about town. After all, they had the serious work of building towns and villages, and their hair said so.

Not all men wanted their hair short, however. Premature balding has always been a problem for men, and during the nineteenth century, as now, some men used longer hair to hide (or disguise) this unwanted change. Corson tells us that

> by the 1840s the neoclassic influence could be seen only on older men who had worn their hair combed forward in their youth and had simply continued to do so, often deliberately, in order to conceal a receding hairline. The hair was usually parted on the side with the side hair brushed straight down, then slightly forward. It tended to be fairly full to the neck in back.[25]

So it seems that men have never liked the idea of losing their hair and exposing their baldness — which may have motivated them to grow (and groom) hair on other visible parts of the body, like the face. Seen as "vulgar, grotesque, and a corrupting influence," wrote Corson, the initial appearance of beards and mustaches during this time was "met with considerable resistance." Regardless, facial hair was popular throughout the nineteenth century and became an issue that prompted men to stand up for their manly rights.[26] Alexander Rowland said,

> Deprive the lion of his mane, the cock of his comb, the pea-cock of the emerald plumage of its tail, the ram and deer of their horns, and they not only become displeasing to the eye, but lose much of their power and vigor . . . The caprice of fashion alone forces the Englishman to shave off those append-ages which give to the male countenance that true masculine character indicative of energy, bold daring, and decision.[27]

Hence, facial hair — a symbol of masculinity — was a way of preserving one's manhood (especially in the face of a receding hair-line). After all, men were given hair to sport their gender and adver-tise their sexuality — or, better said, to strut their stuff.[28] Facial hair on a fighting man had a threefold purpose in history, said Cooper. First, it is — as Darwin said — a badge of sexual maturity, an invita-tion to females. Second, hairiness bolsters the soldier's manhood and virility, an added strength when facing the enemy. Third, it helps to frighten the enemy away (epigamic hair).[29]

Hats (for men) were also popular during the nineteenth century and hid most of their hair (and balding). The hat — especially the top hat — provided a symbol of respectability and a tool with which to flirt.[30] According to Cunnington, tipping one's hat to a lady was a delicate (and rather lewd) compliment. "In his subconscious mind is the barbarous thought that he would gladly take off everything for her sake."[31]

Whiskers, mustaches, hats, and length of hair "waxed and waned" throughout most of the nineteenth century,[32] said Corson, but by the early years of the twentieth century, most men were clean shaven and hair was kept short.[33] As women inched toward freedom, men moved into a formation that looked like an army platoon. During this time in both Europe and the United States, short hair on men was highly valued by many older and middle-aged people. It was a "canon of absolute value,"[34] wrote R. Firth — a style that spoke of an un-questioned willingness to be militant, to conform, to follow the rules, or perhaps it was a reflection of wartime. Men were focused on de-fending their countries (in whatever way they could) against older, more established forces, and they faced this commitment with no-nonsense hair.

Some men, however, did fall prey to the hairstyles of the American movie stars of the 1920s. Rudolph Valentino and George Raft introduced a sleek style, the patent-leather look, and some men liked the pompadour, but men in general, wore their hair "short and neat and that was all."[35] When they could afford to do so (as in between wars), men were a little fussier about their hair, because it turned wavy during the 1930s, and less wavy during the 1940s (during World War II).

When Elvis Presley arrived on the scene in the 1950s, everything changed. Hair, for men, got bigger. The flat-top was popular and so were hair pieces.[36] Elvis was a handsome dude, and his full, dark, sexy hair was part of his appeal. Women were screaming, crying, and fainting at the very sight of this famous songster. The Beatle's mop tops introduced even longer hair in the early 1960s,[37] and mens' hair has never been the same. Like Jake said, "Men start growing their hair long in order to be like the rock stars that women want, and that's one of our prime objectives as males . . . to find women!"

It was quite shocking when men began to wear their hair long. Recognized as a "quasi-political symbol,"[38] it was a "breach of the code of uniformity," a stand against societal norms,[39] wrote Firth. According to Timothy Miller, "Hair was one of the most visible symbols of the culture of opposition . . . Why did hippies grow their hair long? Primarily as a symbol of separateness, or, as Richard Neville put it, 'as a countercultural declaration of independence.' Long hair, beards, no bras and freaky clothes represent a break from Prison Amerika. Indeed, for some time, hippies loved to call themselves freaks."[40]

There is more to the male hippie's long hair, however, than just a symbol of separateness. For years, length of hair has been a gender signifier in Western society. According to Synnott, long hair on the female spoke of femininity and sexuality, sometimes representing spellbinding qualities (such as being able to captivate and manipulate men).[41] Hence, longer hair on men was seen (by some) as a lean toward femininity (an effort to develop their feminine side). This broader interpretation of long hair on men was missed by the larger world, according to Miller, that of the blatant countercultural shift toward androgynous appearance. Regardless, this move toward unity, equality, and wholeness was important, and marked the beginning of a decided change in how men and women relate to one another.[42]

Even today, in some parts of the world, the ways that people wear their hair (especially men) have been "strongly conventionalized," said Firth, sanctioned by an authoritative force, and used to keep certain groups under control.[43] Obvious examples in Western culture are within the armed forces and in prison settings, where a nearly shaved head signifies confinement in an authoritarian environment. Another institution is the home.

Jake, who grew up in the 1970s, said that his father would cut all of his (Jake's) hair off and give him a crew cut and that he "couldn't stand that." He said that his parents were a little rigid, that his father was "pretty much of a control figure." (His dad had attended Catholic schools, a military school, and then embarked on a thirty-year career in the military.) Jake said that he finally rebelled and let his hair grow longer. "I wanted to have my own hair. I had nice, blond, youthful hair, and I wanted to have it — not have it cut off every year."

It is interesting how humans as a species have managed to attach so much power and symbolism to hair. Compared to other parts of the body, however, it isn't too hard to figure out. Our hair is a feathery ornament with which we can express ourselves — a silent emissary, one with a clear and distinct message. And when an individual is losing (or has lost) his or her hair, all of the creative options for making the hair (or social) statement of his or her choice are gone. Mark, who is experiencing male pattern baldness, said, "I think it comes down to options. I think that's what it comes down to for me, is just flat out options." Yolanda agreed. "There's no freedom . . . if you're losing your hair, you're very restricted . . . you feel confined . . . you feel caged."

THE SOCIAL EFFECTS OF HAIR LOSS

We have always known that hair is important, but perhaps not *why*. Simply put, our hair is an instrument that helps us make a statement. Because it can be manipulated in ways that modify our appearance, any change in style or color can significantly alter the perception of who we are or want to be. According to Henry Finck, a new and flattering hair stlye can improve our appearance immediately, and change the way we present ourselves.

If not the most beautiful part of the head, hair certainly is the most beautifying. To improve the shape of mouth, nose, chin, or eyes requires time and patience, but the arrangement of the hair can be altered in a minute, not only to its own advantage, but so as to enhance the beauty of the whole face. By clever manipulation of her long tresses, a woman can alter her appearance almost as completely as a man can by shaving off his long beard or moustache.[44]

For an individual experiencing hair loss, it can be a trying experience facing each day with the challenge of creating a natural and desired appearance, one that represents his or her unique individuality. Hattie, diagnosed with alopecia, says that she gets up in the mornings and says to herself, "What in the world am I gonna do with my hair for the day? So I began to get more and more depressed . . . you know . . . trying to hide it with bobby pins, pulling hair over and stuff."

Daily life is simply more difficult for many people experiencing hair loss. The image that they are forced to present often doesn't match up with who they feel they are. Even wearing a wig is a compromise. Angela said that after she got it [a wig] she wouldn't wear it. "Because it wasn't me . . . it just wasn't me at all." Some say that they feel "different" than their peers, that they "don't fit in." Others report feelings of fear and anxiety, mostly about being rejected, socially and romantically.[45] Psychological research has shown that these feelings are not superficial.

One's physical appearance is, no doubt, the most easily noticeable quality of being human and the one that is most apt to create or affect an impression, especially a first impression. Because hair is a major aspect of one's appearance (as people are almost always physically described by the color and length of their hair, among other identifying qualities), significant hair loss is likely to be noticed right away and filed in the observer's memory, along with feelings and character perceptions about the balding individual. Tom Cash said that

people hold assumptions and attitudes about physical attributes and readily, often nonconsciously, sort people into a variety of cognitive categories or prototypes. These appearance-cued first impressions may act as a funnel, through which other perceptions, expectations, feelings, and social behaviors are channeled. Thus, first impressions persist in the eye of the beholder to the extent that they set the stage for self-confirming, cognitive, and social behavioral processes.[46]

This way of constructing attitudes about others is rather common, but sometimes incorrect and often unfair. Both Jake and Roger said that they felt judged or perceived as not attractive and that the impression they make on others is not accurate. Jake said that living in a society that values physical attributes so much means that you're basically categorized immediately. "Oh, there's some geek! I have received comments from people that were so obvious that they had already categorized me into an intellectual, mature, stable category — before they even said what they did. And they didn't know me at the time."

Roger, too, felt that he was judged unfairly. "I think it is just a shame that the balding male has to be the butt of the joke, that he is not deemed a sexy or attractive man. He is more often seen as nerdy . . . maybe the intellectual."

Indeed, balding males are viewed as older and more intelligent, say Wogalter and Hosie. Research conducted by these two men revealed that balding men do appear older and "also more intelligent (cf. Cash, 1990)." And the results were not surprising; after all, hair loss is generally a sign of aging. The fact that balding men appear to be more intelligent may, perhaps, be linked to the supposition that *older is wiser*.[47]

We do notice hair loss. We are aware of physical differences, we characterize and describe one another's physical make up, and we make assumptions about people based on appearances, probably too much so.

However, some individuals tend to be more focused on themselves when in the presence of others. They worry about how they appear to the group, and this often affects their behavior.[48] This is especially true if an individual is feeling self-conscious about a difference in physical appearance (or perceived flaw), such as hair loss. Bruce said that he felt more sure of himself and was more assertive before he lost his hair.

I used to be a very, very vocal person — very much a type of leader through high school. Through college I was swim team captain . . . group leader of various projects . . . tons of self-confidence. Just very happy with myself. And through the years — I don't know if it's all hair loss . . . I was never afraid of saying how I felt. It [the hair loss] has changed my life in various ways.

Mark said that he doesn't even want to have his picture taken because of his hair loss. "I think that's the first thing people will think of. I think that's how I will be characterized." Joy said that she's careful to hold her head certain ways and not let the car windows down. She said that she didn't want anybody to see (or know) that she was losing her hair. "I don't want it to be shown, and have people ask me about it, or why my hair is missing there. I guess that's what it's all about. I'm just self-conscious about it."

It seems, then, that many balding individuals quietly fret about their appearance and are painfully concerned about the image that they present to the world. These feelings — due to an often impolite and sometimes unforgiving world — may be socially induced. Angela said that she "felt like a freak." She described her hair loss as "patchy bald. I felt like . . . people are looking. And people were looking."

Sheila, who has alopecia universalis (no hair at all on her body), wears a lovely wig and flawless makeup and is one of the most attractive women I have ever met, yet she is rarely comfortable when meeting people. She said that she feels "guarded" when she's with a crowd (especially a new crowd) and that she always anticipates being asked a lot of questions. "Hang on! Eventually they're gonna ask! They're lookin' at ya! They're staring at ya'! They're probably wondering, 'Is that her hair?' It's like all the time, they're gonna ask you. It's coming!"

Thomas, a high-school teacher, keeps his head up high.

I guess in the last few years I've realized that if I'll bend over . . . in other words, to look at me head-on, it's not obvious. But if I bend over, there's more hair loss on top. And I've worked some in the school system, and students can be kind of rough in terms of saying things. And so that's made me more sensitive to the fact that . . . I guess I, in a way, try not to put myself in a compromising situation; put myself where all my baldness is revealed at once, or whatever.

One day at work one of the secretaries noticed a balding area on Hattie's scalp and "made a big deal out of it . . . That really embarrassed me because I had other employees around me, and I only had told one person at work that if she saw a spot that was showing through the hair to act like she was doing something to my hair and push my pin back."

Aside from family members, friends, strangers, students, and co-workers, one of the more unforgiving aspects of modern life is the media. Roger said that it was apparent to him in the business world that for men (as well as women) images and impressions are very important.

> We are constantly bombarded with commercials on TV about the way we look. And, so I am definitely aware and wondering what other people think of me and my image. Do they like me because I look a certain way? Mostly, I think about how they will perceive me in comparison to other people. You know, how many times do you see a young, bald male as a sexy model?

And when Walt was checking out options for treating his hair loss he discovered that people try to "sell you what you couldn't get when you were young."

> They pound it into you . . . this is how you're supposed to look, and you're supposed to be cool, and you're supposed to be suave, and it's normal for women to fawn over you. And you're supposed to look like all the guys on soap operas. It's just like women who get bombarded with images of Playboy bunnies and that sort of thing . . . it really is a traumatic thing. And it's the same sort of thing that women experience with aging.

Hence, many individuals experiencing hair loss feel that they don't measure up. They feel different. Expressed as a feeling of not belonging — the difference that they experience affects their social interactions, feelings of self-worth, and beliefs about their physical attractiveness.[49] When Sheila was reflecting on her teenage years, she said that she wouldn't go to parties or hang out with a crowd. "I didn't like to be around groups of people. Everything is changing. Here you are, fifteen or sixteen years old, and all of a sudden everybody is getting asked out. I never really dated anybody. I was ashamed. I felt ashamed because I was different."

Bret said that he, too, felt out of place when he was in a crowd of people, male or female.

> In situations like being in a class full of other people, you know ... it would tend to make me a little quieter, or a little more self-conscious than I normally would have been ... just the feeling of being different ... and therefore people are looking at you because you're not fitting into the crowd or something.

Don seemed to feel that he was excluded not only from mixed groups but also from groups of males.

> When you're younger, groups are formed a lot of times on popularity ... your own attractiveness or whatever ... and it just kinda makes me feel like you're out of groups just simply because of your appearance, which you had no control over. If baldness is the problem, you were predisposed. Good-looking guys will, a lot of times, be with other good-looking guys. And if there's a kind of attitude in society that being bald is not attractive, then you may worry that you're gonna be precluded from some groups because they're gonna be worried that being with you makes them seem less attractive or something ... I've seen that enough times in my life.

Roger enjoyed a full head of hair all through high school, then experienced rapid hair loss the summer before attending his state university.

> Here I was, a young man who had always had long hair, was very interested in having it styled in the latest fashion, was very concerned with his appearance. I went from being on

the top of the hill in high school to feeling, "Oh, gee, I'm on the bottom of the pool here."

Physical attractiveness is important, particularly in dating behavior. Studies indicate that not only is it helpful to be attractive but it is gratifying to be with (i.e., to date) someone who is physically appealing.[50] Hence, people who are experiencing hair loss and believe that they are physically unattractive tend to feel insecure in the dating arena. Jake said that all through high school he hadn't participated much and hadn't had a large group of friends. "I was hoping that college would be something different. And, of course, you want to date women. And you're out of the game if you are a freshman with a receding hairline. And the scene that you're in as a freshman in college . . . it's all physical for the most part."

Helen said that she had a fear that stemmed from rejection fantasies. "I've been a single person my whole life, and it [hair loss] didn't alter my feeling of fear of rejection . . . and growing old alone . . . and all of those feelings that I don't think are terribly uncommon."

And so it goes, the emotional fragility and overwhelming sensitivity that accompanies hair loss. "It is so emotional," said Brad.

It is so emotionally charged. It's something that happens, that is not recognized as a problem, even a medical problem. You're not going to go talk to your buddy about it. People are not going to make an appointment to talk to their therapist about their hair loss. It's something that's just not recognized. You deal with it on a personal level.

So, generally speaking, they don't talk about it. The fear of being thought of as vain or shallow or of being misunderstood forces individuals experiencing hair loss to be alone with their feelings and vulnerable to thoughtless comments. Many struggle in social situations and with society in general. Living in a culture that holds youth and physical attractiveness in such high esteem makes it all the more difficult.

Hence, many people experiencing hair loss carry around invisible emotional wounds. Some feel excluded, teased, categorized, and judged; some fear rejection (especially by the opposite sex); many feel different than their peers. "Well," said Don, "you kinda feel like this from looking around at what is reinforced in society. Every model, every star, everybody pretty much . . . they have hair."

⌐

Hair is a powerful symbol of one's individuality. It is a part of the body that we can be creative with, a way of projecting who we are. Yet, hair can have social as well as personal significance, as hairstyles have not always been a matter of personal choice. In centuries past in Europe and in the United States, hairstyles revealed a good bit about social mores and societal expectations (which varied according to gender, age, and marital and financial status).

So the history of both mens' and womens' hairstyles tells an interesting story of a steady progression toward equality and a more liberal society. Over time, in Western society, the various ways people wore their hair became clear personal statements, and eventually, a sign of rebellion or anti-establishment views.

It's a different way of life, however, for people who are losing their hair. For many, it is an emotionally complicated experience that involves more than concern about body image. There seems to be a level of discomfort, largely due to a feeling of not living up to society's expectations to remain young and attractive. Many fear rejection (especially by the opposite sex), some feel different than their peers. Above all, many feel that they cannot portray an image that best represents who they are. Furthermore, these individuals seem to have little or no emotional support for the feelings they experience as a result of losing their hair. Men are teased about going bald, and women are criticized for being vain. Hence, the experience of losing one's hair can result in feelings of isolation, insecurity, and self-doubt (especially in social situations), which are magnified by an unforgiving and insensitive world and by the media.

CHAPTER THREE

RAPUNZEL, RAPUNZEL . . .

The Unconscious Meaning of Hair

CONSCIOUS ACT (UNCONSCIOUS PUPOSE)

Sally was 20 years old when she was married. She was young, but girls married young back then, usually right after high school. A devout Catholic, she began to have a baby every year, eventually giving birth to seven children: five

All of this may teach us nothing more than we have already suspected, namely that our hair activities are but another substitutive expression of our sexual conflict — conspicuously a genital level of conflict.

— Charles Berg

sons and two daughters. At first there were only boys in her growing family, four of them. Then Sara arrived: the first girl born into her husband's established, well-to-do family in three generations, and everyone was pretty happy about it — everyone but Katherine, Sally's mother-in-law. Katherine, who lived one block away, had been the only woman in the clan until Sally married her son, and she seemed to have liked that role. Sally understood this. So when Sara was born, Katherine wasn't particularly thrilled about it. Katherine was slowly losing her status as the special female in the family — a fact that she was aware of more than anyone else — and everyone simply tiptoed around her feelings.

Sally was later divorced (again at a young age), an event that in this small Catholic community was unheard of. It caused a great deal of gossip and unpleasantness, and immediately severed the relationship between Sally and her in-laws. She eventually moved to a small town on the west coast of Florida, mainly to create privacy for herself and her children. After that the children saw their father and grandparents during the summer months and over long holiday vacations.

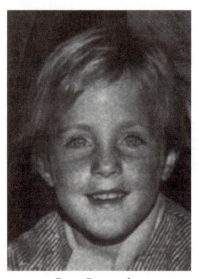

Sara Romweber
Christmas, 1969.

Six months after the move to Florida, the children were spending Christmas vacation with their dad and grandparents at a lovely resort on the east coast. The children looked good. They were tan, their hair was blond from living in a year-round sunny climate, and they were healthy. Sara, now about five years old, had beautiful, long, golden hair. But when she returned from her Christmas visit, she didn't have it any longer. Her lovely, long hair had been cut off. According to Sara, her grandmother took her to a beautician in the hotel.

Sara seemed unaffected by her haircut, but Sally was stunned. The other children had longer hair, and Katherine didn't opt to change that. Only years later did the meaning of this willful deed become apparent. Sara was the apple of her dad's (and grandfather's) eye, and she was named after her mother. ("Sally" is a nickname for Sara.) The act of cutting Sara's hair was Katherine's way of defeminizing the women who had stolen the hearts of her men. It was a symbolic act, one with an unconscious purpose, and a desire to punish.

THE UNCONSCIOUS MIND

For the purposes of this chapter, the word unconscious refers to that part of the psyche (or mind) that is not readily available to one's consciousness or state of awareness. For example, much of our dreaming is believed to take place in an unconscious state. One does not have to be asleep, however, to have activity going on in the unconscious mind. The unconscious is an active part of the psyche, and it churns out bits and pieces of information throughout the day — such as slips of the tongue (accidentally using the word funeral for the word wedding) and other surprising behaviors. Most of us have heard someone say, "I don't know why I did that [or said that], it just happened."

When we speak of the unconscious mind we tend to think of Sigmund Freud, largely because this was the primary focus of his work. Freud used the analogy of an iceberg to describe what he believed to be the three states of mind: the conscious, the preconscious, and the unconscious. The conscious mind is compared to that section of the iceberg that is above water (that which we are aware of). The preconscious mind is compared to the large chunk of ice just below the surface of the water; it holds the thoughts and images that we are not aware of all the time but can bring into our consciousness at will. Freud compared the unconscious to that enormous part of the iceberg that lies well below the surface of the water, clearly illustrating that this is a part of the mind that is buried deep within the psyche — below one's level of awareness.[1]

Freud's work became known as psychoanalytic theory or psychoanalysis. This theory places major emphasis on (1) the psychosexual development of human beings, (2) the unconscious aspects of the personality, and (3) the use of symbols (images or words that mean something else). His theory also suggests that many of our conscious thoughts and actions (those we are aware of) are caused by repressed feelings, attitudes, and conflicts (those which we are not aware of); that words, feelings, attitudes, and conflicts too overwhelming or unacceptable for us to deal with consciously are buried deep in the unconscious. These feelings and attitudes do, however — as mentioned earlier — emerge in such behaviors as dreaming, slips of the tongue, and other unexplained urges.[2] In other words, repressed feelings and urges that are often sexual are believed to manifest in everyday life in hidden ways, such as saying, "Please pass the black peter," when one really means to say, "Please pass the black pepper." Another common manifestation of sexual repression is the use of the word bondage, instead of bonding, which most of us have read (or heard) a time or two.

Many of the psychological treatments or techniques used in psychoanalysis require superb interpretive skills on the part of the therapist, mainly because behaviors — such as unacceptable thoughts or bizarre dreams — presented by the client are believed to be complicated, as well as symbolic, and require an ability (on the part of the therapist) to make sense of it all. Hence, one premise of psychoanalytic thought is that all behavior has meaning and much of the time this meaning is hidden from the individual demonstrating it (the client). However, through psychoanalysis — which generally involves years of therapy — a client can begin to understand the meaning of his or her thoughts, urges, and other such behaviors.

THE UNCONSCIOUS MEANING OF HAIR

Symbols — the use of sophisticated thoughts or images in place of something else — are important in psychoanalysis. For example, most of us are familiar with the notion of phallic symbols (images that resemble the penis), such as a skyscrapers, cigars or any long, pointy objects. Now let's talk about hair.

According to psychoanalytic theory, the hair on the head is sexually symbolic. Charles Berg, a well-known psychoanalyst, said that the hair is "conspicuously a genital [sexual] symbol" and that "our mental attitude towards hair and our activities with it are a displaced expression of our sexual conflict (at the genital level)." He maintained that the sexual significance of hair is buried in the subconscious mind, a result of having lived in a civilized world, and people use their hair to express sexual feelings because it is "a convenient and suitable symbol for the repressed tension of the unconscious [sexual] conflict."[3] In other words, our Puritan heritage, which preached that sex is wrong and dirty, motivated us to repress our natural feelings and urges about sexual activity and made those thoughts unacceptable in the conscious mind. Berg suggests that fooling around with one's hair is a covert way of acting out our repressed sexual feelings.

No one can deny that there are casual and unconscious uses of the hair that appear to be sexual. As mentioned previously, tossing the head to flip the hair out of one's face is a flirting (or sexual) gesture. More to the point, when a woman plays with her hair (when in a crowd

and mingling), it's a covert way of saying that she can be touched.
Berg's theory about the symbolism of hair has been the subject
of much opposition (as well as praise). It is illustrated as follows:

head = phallus (penis)
hair = semen
hair cutting = castration (removal of hormone-producing sex organs)[4]

RAPUNZEL AND THE THEME OF CASTRATION

Most of us are all familiar with the fairy tale of Rapunzel.
Rapunzel is a young girl held prisoner in a tower by an enchantress
in a large forest. She has very long, beautiful hair, which she lowers
through a window at the top of the tower. The enchantress visits
Rapunzel by climbing up the long golden braid. One day Rapunzel is
surprised by a different visitor — a prince, who has been secretly
watching the tower and the visiting enchantress. Rapunzel allows
the prince to climb into the tower (via her braid) and visit with her.
The prince, of course, falls in love with her, proposes marriage, and
plans her escape from the tower. The enchantress, however, learns of
their plans. She cuts Rapunzel's beautiful, long hair; removes her
from the tower; and hides her in the desert. The enchantress then
returns to the tower (with Rapunzel's hair) to wait for the prince.
The prince comes to visit Rapunzel, shinnies up the braid, and finds
the enchantress waiting for him in the tower. The prince is brutally
punished by the enchantress for trying to take Rapunzel away.[5]

In an article titled "Rapunzel: The Symbolism of the Cutting of
Hair," J. J. Andresen, a psychoanalyst, offers several interpretations
of cutting Rapunzel's hair — one being that it is a form of castration.
For a female this is believed to mean the removal of the ability to
enjoy sex. Andresen said that when the enchantress cut Rapunzel's
braid, Rapunzel no longer has a way to visit with the prince and,
consequently, was unable to have a lover (or sexual relationship).
And without her hair, she was no longer desirable or appealing to the
opposite sex.[6] One version of the story is that the prince is blinded by
the enchantress when he climbs into the tower. He and Rapunzel
eventually find each other in the woods, still love one another, and

begin a new life together, meaning, perhaps, that the only lover she can have, is one who is blind to her imperfection.

Andresen said that he reached his conclusion about the symbolism of Rapunzel's shorn hair through the interpretation of dreams reported by four of his female patients. The dreams were all about haircuts, which, he said, coexisted with fears of physical unattractiveness or defectiveness.[7]

Several of the women that I spoke with indicated that Andresen's theory is correct. They had all lost (or were losing) their hair, and all spoke about feeling sexually undesirable. Yolanda seemed to feel as if she were damaged goods. "I didn't want anybody to know I was going bald. I was in my thirties, had four children, wanted to be married again. I don't want to be by myself the rest of my life."

Grace said that during her hair loss experience, her husband kept his distance from her. "I kind of felt like it was going to be a long time before I felt really attractive to him." Sheila acknowledges that her lack of a relationship may well be due to her hair loss and her own feelings about it.

Sadly, these perceptions may be objectively accurate. Several years ago, while attending a holiday brunch, the subject of my research came up. All of the guests were seated around a large table, enjoying great food, and the men began teasing one another about losing their hair. The host spoke sorrowfully about the time his wife (who was listening to the discussion) had cut her hair quite short — apparently without warning him first. "It took me weeks to get over it," he said. You could tell that it was a sensitive subject when their 30-year-old son became a little nervous. "I felt so bad for mom. I told her that it looked good. I tried to be supportive."

Men, too, seem to feel somewhat defiled when their hair is cut too short. Kevin, a handsome young man who was attending the brunch — he had beautiful, shoulder-length hair — told us of his fierce opposition to having his hair cut when he was a little boy. "It felt like I was being violated ... like being circumcised in public." He went to the barber 'kicking and screaming!" According to Andresen, a severe haircut (or loss of hair) symbolizes castration for men as well (a feeling reported by one of his male patients).

A story similar to Kevin's was told by a friend of mine in graduate school. She said that her husband's son (an adolescent) had wanted to wear his hair long. Long hair was apparently fine with his stepmom and dad, but it soon became a problem when he didn't wash or comb it. It became tangled and matted, no one could get a comb through it, and the only way to solve the problem was to have his hair cut (which the boy didn't want, and which created a new and different problem). He was so upset that for weeks he wore a towel wrapped around his head. He wouldn't even come out of his room.

Another psychoanalyst, M. D. Eder, reported a theory similar to Andresen's when he spoke of a female client who was in anguish over the prospects of having her hair cut. Eder said that his client scheduled and canceled many appointments to have her hair styled in a short, layered cut, or "shingled." She finally did go to her appointment, but as soon as the first strand of hair was cut, she became ill and nearly fainted. She said that after some smelling salts she agreed to continue with the cutting and styling, and that she finally made it through the procedure. However, she told Eder that she felt faint and dizzy the rest of the day. Then she reported a dream that she had the night before her hair appointment. She said that she was in a large bath of water alone with her little son, and that he slipped under the water. Regardless of her efforts and screams for help she couldn't rescue him. She said that it was the worst nightmare she ever had; she woke up terrified, bathed in sweat, and certain that her little boy had drowned. Eder interpreted the loss of the boy (in the dream) as a fear of castration — his client's fear of losing her sexuality.[8]

Getting one's hair cut can feel a little scary, but even just damage to the hair can be traumatic. Any hairstylist will tell you that customers (particularly women) are inclined to get upset — even cry — if their hair is unintentionally cut too short or ruined in any way.

Responses to Psychoanalytic Theory About the Unconscious Meaning of Hair

To some theorists, psychoanalytic notions about hair are absurd — especially the idea of one's head symbolizing a penis and hair representing semen. Even well-known theorists who say that hair is used extensively in ritual behavior in various cultures (and is symbolic worldwide) have a problem with the unconscious meaning that psychoanalysts attribute to hair. They say that in many cultures there is a sexual meaning associated with hair, but they don't see this as particularly important. For example, E. R. Leach says that Berg has overgeneralized the notion of hair being sexual as an "unconscious" act, and he gives some critical examples of conscious uses of harsh haircuts as sexual statements. He discusses the rigorous celibacy imposed on Hindu widows — the requirement that they shave their heads as an expression of a new station in life (do not have sexual partners). He speaks about the common practice of Buddhist monks and nuns (celibate individuals) shaving their heads, while people who lead normal sex lives have hair (sometimes wearing it long).[9]

Leach sees a problem with the meaning psychoanalysts attribute to hair, stating that they use "anthropological materials to support conclusions of a psychoanalytic kind." He writes that "hairdressing is an extremely widespread feature of ritual behavior ... a universal symbol ... and not specifically a sexual one."[10] He acknowledges that hair rituals may have sexual associations, but says this is not regarded as critical.

Leach explains, as does M. Douglas,[11] that ritual behavior is primarily "a form of communication"[12] and that the symbols used have a common meaning for everyone involved. His objection to Berg's statements is his overgeneralization that

> some modern neurotic patients "repress into the unconscious" all recognition of any association between the head of the body and the head of the phallus; from this he infers that all ordinary members of our society do this — unless they have the benefit of psychoanalysis, and that, by contrast, all primitive savages are free of this sickness of civilization.[13]

Both Leach and Douglas propose that hair symbolism simply transmits something about the culture and is not buried in the subconscious.

However, in defense of psychoanalytic theory, Leach seems to understand the sexual symbolism of hair within various cultures. What isn't clear is whether or not the individuals involved in the particular cultural norms do. In other words, the sexual association with hair may (or may not be) an unconscious act for those involved. Another theorist, P. Hershman, explains my point a little better in his report on Sikh Punjabi hairdressing.

THE SIKH RITUALS OF HAIRDRESSING

Hershman, who spent time with Sikh Punjabi societies (located in northern India) and observed their daily rituals, gives an impressive account of the attitudes and beliefs involving hair among these people — and he strongly suggests that these beliefs gain their power through an unconscious connection with the genital organs. Hershman's observations — which focused mainly on the culture's grooming, language, religious practices, and verbal communication — reveal a level of repressed sexual conflict which manifest in rituals with hair.[14]

> It is my hypothesis that in its symbolic usage hair gains its power through its equivalence with the genital organs in the individual Punjabi subconscious but that it is then culturally employed in ritual, in co-ordination with other symbols, as a means of communicating certain essential values of Punjabi society.[15]

Hershman said that in Punjabi society hair grooming is performed in private; that grooming another person's hair is considered an intimate act and carries with it strong sexual undertones. For example, a Punjabi male may have his hair cut by a barber, but the grooming (i.e., washing, combing) is always done by a woman. It is never performed by a sister to her brother (unless he is very young), and it is not a service provided by one man to another. It is a service provided by a woman to her husband. Women, however, do groom one anothers' hair — a ritual that is performed reciprocally between female relatives. Furthermore, it is important for the female to have long, healthy hair (and for the males to retain their hair).

> Whereas the removal of body hair is thought to be sexually enhancing, Punjabi women believe that the longer they grow the head hair the more sexually attractive they become, and similarly Punjabi men see their sexual decline in balding or greying hair and many attempt to arrest this process by dyeing their sparse hair red or black.[16]

Punjabis who live by the strict rules of the Sikh religion never cut their hair, so without proper grooming it can become quite tangled and dirty. The grooming process is intense and sensual. It involves: (1) careful washing of the hair in buttermilk; (2) thorough drying; (3) an oil application; (4) combing to remove tangles (a painful procedure); and (5) pulling the hair tightly together, toward the back, in a knot or braid. This grooming process gives both pain and pleasure to another, and, according to Hershman, "reveals a clear connection between sexuality and grooming." Consistent with psychoanalytic thought, Hershman believes that the sexual feelings related to grooming the hair are suppressed in the unconscious.[17]

The Punjabi culture is a very sexually repressed culture, a fact that is evident in their language. Sex is a forbidden topic of conversation. The sexual organs are never mentioned (except when swearing), and the word for hair, val, is rarely used because it refers to the pubic hair. Instead of saying val, the Punjabis use the word syr (meaning head), and the Sikhs use the word *kes*, which is a special ritual word for the head hair. Hershman said that in the unconscious minds of the Punjabis, the head is identified with the sexual organ [the penis] but that it is the hair which is symbolic of its emissions and sexuality in general; which is the exact symbolism that Berg described. Hershman said that the Sikh Punjabis prefer to use the term for head rather than use the word for hair "because it is not the genitals which are in themselves obscene but only the sexuality associated with them."[18]

Within the Punjabi culture, the sexual association with hair is most apparent in one particular ceremony. As mentioned earlier, the Punjabi women generally do not cut their hair. They wear it parted in the middle, with the sides pulled tightly toward the back into braids. In certain rituals — such as in a high-caste Hindu marriage ceremony — the central parting of the hair is reddened. According to Hershman, the smearing of red in the hair parting is a symbol of the vagina and "more concretely of vaginal and menstrual blood."[19]

> Only a woman whose husband is alive may redden this parting with vermilion, and a part of the high caste Hindu marriage ceremony amongst some clans is for the groom to smear a little vermilion into his bride's hair parting.[20]

The symbolism of hair in the Sikh Punjabi society (on an individual subconscious level) seems to be the notion of keeping sexual energy under control. Hershman said that between the two levels of symbolism — the cultural and the subconscious — "there is a strong connecting element in the belief of Punjabis that controlled sexuality is the source of spiritual power."[21]

Because the meaning of a symbol is generally the work of the subconscious mind, and because subconscious activity is relatively similar to all of humankind (and generally related to sexual repression), there are several theories offered for what the exact use of hair as a cultural symbol might mean. The first is that which relates to sex or sexual impulses — that used by the Sikh Punjabis — which, of course, is the energy that propels us to produce offspring (the libido), perpetuate life (the life force), and survive as a species. The second way of using hair as a cultural symbol may simply be a particular group's way of organizing their world — meanings that may have a sexual basis and may also be unconscious.

THE POWHATANS' USE OF HAIRDRESSING

The Powhatan Indians (a tribe discovered by the Jamestown Colony in the early 1600s) are a good example of how hair was used as a means of organizing their society (or world). This group was predominantly known for the hairstyle worn by the male commoners: an asymmetrical hairstyle (long on the left, and short on the right). The tribe (allegedly) reported that short hair on the right side of the head kept it from getting caught in bowstrings. Margaret Williamson, however, suggests that this is an "exegetical explanation," or too simple an interpretation.

> It is practical and even obvious. But it does not explain why the other side of the head was not so shorn; and on closer examination we find that it is not even a necessary reason for cutting the hair on the right since a similar effect could be gained by binding the hair back.[22]

The asymmetrical hairstyle worn by the Powhatan men "is but one of a great many expressions of the basic assumptions according to which the Powhatan" organized the world, wrote Williamson.[23]

There were two reasons for this particular hairstyle, one being that it was obviously practical. However, before we look further into this famous hairstyle we need to examine all of the hairstyles worn by the tribal members, because there was a particular style worn by each of the Powhatans and each hairstyle had a special meaning.

- Shamans: The shamans were the religious leaders. They were known as the medicine men. Their heads were almost entirely shaven. The shamans were always male. They did not grow gardens and they did not have children. The shaman was the highest ranking member of the tribe.

- Werowances: The werowances were the chiefs, and they were ranked between the shaman and the male commoner. Their heads were shaven, but a headdress was worn. This headdress was somewhat like a crown. It was partially made of deers' hair (colored red) which circled the left, and the right side of the crown was decorated with a copper plate. The chief had qualities of both the shaman and a male commoner. He knew more about the tribal secrets and religious mystic than the commoner, but he was allowed to have a wife and children (and grow a garden). His role was to serve as a mediator for his people with outsiders.

- Females: The adult females wore their hair long. They had children and they grew gardens.

- Commoner: The commoners were male. They wore asymmetric hairstyles. The hair on the left side of the head was long (sometimes 45 inches in length), rolled up into a knot and held in place with an ornament such as a long feather. The hair on the right was shaven.

The reason for the asymmetric hair style worn by the male commoners was that these men considered themselves to be both male and female. They viewed the right side of the body (the side with the short hair) as masculine, and the left side (the side with the long hair) as feminine. The thinking behind this had something to do with their activities, or the division of their labors. They were the hunters, which was a male activity (short hair on the right). Yet they were also involved with family and tending crops, which were female activities (long hair on the left). In other words, the commoners —

who were ordinary men — dealt with death (hunting) and with life (producing children, growing crops). The chart below presents more clearly the significance of the Powhatan hairstyles:

Shaman (shaven)

werowance (shaven/headdress/often bearded)

male commoner (asymmetric haircut)

woman (long hair)[24]

The shaman was, in a social sense, considered dead and asexual.[25] He didn't have children, he didn't produce crops, and he didn't have hair. The werowance (considered to be both male and female) "alone grew beards," and "beards are particularly masculine."[26] It's interesting to note, too, that young, unmarried girls wore their hair long in the back, but short in the front and on the sides. This meant that they had no babies — not yet sexually active — and no gardens (short hair in front), but the potential was there to bear children and to grow crops (long hair in back).[27] As previously mentioned, all of the Powhatan hairstyles were symbolic. Each hairstyle endorsed a particular energy that either moved with, or away from, the life force. Furthermore, wearing the correct hairstyle was expected. It was the daily ritual of membership.

The Cultural (and Sometimes Unconscious) Expectations of Hairstyle

"That hair is significant is undeniable," wrote Williamson. "Virtually every society attaches significance to head hair at least."[28] For example, within the continent of Africa, hair is important socially and spiritually and can also have sexual connotations. In this part of the world, certain hairstyles can say something about one's maturity or status in life (social). And certain styles — particularly on young girls — can be a badge of readiness for a relationship with the opposite sex (sexual).[29]

In Nigeria (tropical West Africa), a young woman historically changed her hairstyle as an announcement of maturing. According to Esi Sagay,

As soon as a girl's breasts began to develop she started to dress her hair with the intention of attracting the attention of men. Over a span of eight years she adopted a new style annually, each designed to display her charm and vanity. A particularly beautiful coiffure marked the day of her marriage.[30]

In the Malagasy Republic, women used elegantly designed hair to attract men. In this part of Africa a woman shaved her head if she were widowed.[31] And in North Africa, a — wore three different hairstyles throughout her lifetime: one indicating childhood, one indicating adolescence, and one indicating adulthood. From birth until the age of twelve, her head was partly shaven and the remaining hair was braided (asexual?). During the adolescent years her hair was permitted to grow all over her head and braided into a simple style (pubescent?). The adult women of this culture wore elaborate and complex hairstyles (sexual?). For ceremonial occasions they adorned these hairstyles with ornaments, such as shells and coins.[32]

One cannot say with certainty what hair symbolizes within a particular culture. It may be that within a certain society, hair represents (at an unconscious level) semen, along with the head representing the phallus. It may be that, because it is a highly visible part of the body and can be altered temporarily, hair represents the temporary stages of an individual's life, consciously or unconsciously. [33]

The purpose of this writing is to demonstrate the cultural importance of having a nice head of hair. Hair has a rich history in the world of symbolism. It is, perhaps, used very little (if at all) in rituals and ceremonies around the world any longer, but over the centuries, hair has played an important and historical role in symbolic expression. To explore the symbolism of hair in all cultures of the world would require another book. The purpose of this writing is simply to demonstrate how hair is (or has been) used symbolically — consciously and unconsciously — in several cultures (or groups within a particular culture). Whether the meaning of hair is conscious or unconscious is quite interesting, but inconsequential to my investigation. In most societies it is simply important to have hair. Hair — whether associated with prepubescence, fertility, generation, widowhood, femininity, masculinity, or the sexual organs — is a culturally important part of the body.

The theory that human beings subconsciously (1) see the head as symbolic of a penis, and (2) substitute semen for the cranial hair, appears to be a tribute to Freudian emphasis on repressed sexuality, has no basis in fact, and limits subconscious thought about hair to our sexual nature and the reproductive organs. It feeds the notion that human beings are obsessed with sexual thinking whether they know it or not. This idea is also evident in the proposed "fear of castration" symbol of hair cutting, an interpretation resulting primarily from dream analysis. Could not the cutting of hair in dreams simply represent a sense of powerlessness about certain events in one's life?

Leach's position on the symbolism of head hair does not entirely disclaim psychoanalytic theory, but it does represent a more wholistic approach. Leach says the general feeling among anthropologists is that "hair stands for the total individual or for the soul, or for the individual's power (mana)." He maintains that hair is used in ritual (universally) because it reflects "the progression of the individual through set states in the social system," stages which "correspond to different degrees of maturity, different types of permitted sexual behavior, different allocations of social power." He says that ethnography suggests a "link between hair as a symbol and the phallus as a symbol," and that "to this extent it is appropriate that hair should be prominent in rites denoting a change in social-sexual status."[34]

Sex — one of the two pleasurable urges we are born with (the other being a desire to consume food) — is on our minds consciously and unconsciously. According to the psychoanalytic community, sexual notions manifest in various, seemingly nonsexual human behaviors. It is believed by many theorists that hair activities are an example of how this happens.

Many of us know that a sexual association with hair is not necessarily unconscious. Most of the individuals that I interviewed spoke repeatedly about the sexual importance of hair. Yet, many individuals are quite surprised to learn that hair is a sensual part of the body (which, of course, supports psychoanalytic theory).

CHAPTER FOUR

CROWN AND GLORY

Religious Beliefs and the Matter of Hair

MARRIAGES MADE IN HEAVEN

I watched an interesting TV mini-series several years ago about three young Catholic women who wanted to become nuns. The setting was in Australia, and the time must have been somewhere around the mid-1950s because there was no mention of World War II and it was

> *That same nun insisted we wear hats in church. Quoting St. Paul, she told us that woman, as the instrument of man's downfall in Eden, wasn't fit to appear bareheaded in the house of the Lord.*
>
> — Geraldine Brooks

before the gathering of the second Vatican Council, which took place in the 1960s. The young women didn't know one another, but once inside the abbey they became acquainted and eventually became friends.

These three young women were inexperienced and naive. Whatever sense of self they possessed on the day they entered the convent was quickly snatched away by a strict code of obedience and the daily rigors of religious life. They scrubbed floors, worked in the garden, made endless novenas, sang matins and vespers, recited litanies, and deprived themselves of simple pleasures. Some of the older, more embittered nuns were harsh and unforgiving and made life miserable for the young women. As time passed, they became docile and serene.

During this preparatory stage the girls wore simple, dark clothing, and they all dressed alike. They wore dark shoes and dark stockings; their blouses had long sleeves, and the hems of their skirts were longer than was stylish for that time. Each wore a veil that appeared to be fastened to a headband so that it wouldn't fall off. It covered the hair somewhat, but not entirely.

Some months later, the ones regarded as sufficiently prepared were selected to take their first (temporary) vows, a service which began with the young women entering the chapel in long white gowns. They were bridal gowns, actually, as these young women were believed to be brides of Christ. Toward the end of the ceremony, each young bride ascended the altar and received a neatly folded bundle of clothing — the habit. Then, assembled in single file, they were led by one of the head sisters to a room connected to the chapel.

In the adjacent room the white gowns and bridal veils fell to the floor, and generous amounts of dark, heavy fabric were thrown over frail, upright bodies. Then the viewers hear a loud snip — and watch a beautiful, long, dark braid being tossed casually into a large basket. Handfuls of lovely locks and braids are thrown, one after the other, into large wicker containers. We see startled faces and baskets filled with human hair. We hear sounds of cutting and snipping, and the thrust of hair landing in the crypts — an ancient custom with a powerful message: if one gives herself over to Christ, her hair must be sheared, and her head covered forever.[1]

Better described as a rule than a custom, this treatment of women's hair was historically prevalent in many religious groups. Married Jewish women at one time were required to cover their hair, many Muslim women are still veiled from head to toe, and as our story reminds us, until the mid-1960s Catholic nuns were required to have their hair clipped close to the scalp, sometimes shaved. All but the face was covered with a veil, coif, and a specifically designed (sometimes cumbersome) headdress that identified the order of nuns. Even lay Catholic women were required to cover their hair with a hat, scarf, or veil when attending church services.[2] I can still remember my dear (and very upset) grandmother frantically throwing a handkerchief over my adolescent head as we climbed the church steps one Sunday morning.

In years past — and in some cases still today — synagogue, temple, and church groups all over the world have honored their religious sect's views about covering hair. Some admonish that a woman's hair is alluring — and therefore tempting — to all men and insist that her head be covered when outside the home, or at the very least when attending religious services; saying that it is the law of God or Allah. Ancient tribes in faraway lands view hair as a sacred abode for their personal god, but other more controversial worshippers — those practicing voodoo,[3] witchcraft, or demonology[4] — view hair as a part of the body that holds the soul (or energy) of that particular individual, dead or alive. As you will soon be reminded, hair has a rich history in the world of religious and spiritual symbolism.

Judaism and the Matter of Hair Covering

According to Susan Schneider, "Covered hair was at one time the most observably 'Jewish' part of a woman's appearance." In fact, one of the marks of a married, Jewish female was to have her hair completely covered when she was in public. It had something to do with modesty and morality and the forbidding of provocative, flirtatious dress — all part of a rule (for Jewish women) about not parading one's sexuality in public. This rule, which is no longer exercised in most of Western society, has been interpreted in several ways. Some view the custom of wearing a wig (*sheytl*) or scarf as a religious symbol, believing that covered hair exemplified a more religious or devout way of life, a badge of Jewish identity. There was also the equality factor: the idea that it was simply nice for Jewish women to have a head covering when in synagogue, just as the Jewish men wore a skull cap (*kippah*). Others, however, believe that it had more to do with enhancing dignity, holding to the notion that a Jewish woman should always present herself as reserved and composed (not outwardly expressing sexual desire or prowess).[5] Hence, in Eastern Europe, all married Jewish women historically covered their hair in public. Exposed hair was equal to nudity, similar to undressing in public, tempting and titillating to men, sexually enticing. A married, "bare-headed" Jewish female in public view was considered brazen, portraying herself as a sex object or a male plaything. Appearing in public without a head covering was perceived as flouting one's marriage vows. In fact, the husband could be ordered to divorce this shameless hussy.[6]

It was different behind closed doors, however. Within the confines of marriage and family, a Jewish wife and mother could remove her scarf or wig (her honor) and permit her hair to breathe. At home she could temporarily free herself of an inconvenient custom. Her hair belonged to her husband and children — a tradition that was believed to add a depth and richness to married life and family life. In spite of all the inconvenience, this practice was revered among Jewish women for a time in history.[7]

According to Leo Trepp, the ritual of cutting the hair and covering the head of a Jewish woman traditionally took place before the wedding. He notes:

> As the wedding day approached, showers were given for the bride-to-be. At this occasion, the girl's hair might be cropped. The reason? The faithful woman does not show her hair; only wantons do so (based on Num. 5:18). The Rabbis had also stated that a woman's hair is "nakedness," which only her husband was to see. From now on her hair was covered with a cap.[8]

(As Jewish women ventured out into the world, the cap was replaced with a wig, and nowadays the custom of head covering is observed only "in worship and when lighting the Sabbath candles.)[9]

Because hair has a sensual and provocative quality, leaving it exposed to public view was seen within the Jewish community as a threat to family and social structure. Keeping it covered was a symbol of restraint and self-control for the married female — and also for her public. It was an announcement: Covering the hair protected the sanctity of marriage, family, and the Jewish way of life, a practice that must have sent a powerful message to the children in the family.[10]

As a religious symbol, the wearing of a scarf or *shetyl* may have said, "I am a Jew." But for many Jewish women, it signified more than just a spiritual commitment. For some, the act of head covering appears to have also expressed something of a personal nature. Giti Bendheim, a psychologist, remarks,

> Ultimately, for me, the issue boils down to my own sense of humbleness in the face of an ancient tradition. There is a part

of me that values hair-covering as an act of faith I share with tens of generations of Jewish women before me. After all, covering one's hair is one of the few observances that can be performed only by women. Like the laws of family purity, its observance links me to a whole tradition of Jewish women in the powerful way that only a concrete observance can.[11]

For Jewish women, the act of hair covering appears to have had both an inner — and outer — directed quality of spirituality. It spoke to the inner core ("I embrace my Jewish heritage"), and visually, it spoke to the world. It had a controlling effect on the self ("I'll behave like a lady"), and also on the behavior of others. Hence, it enabled a Jewish female to be more mindful or cognizant of the messages she was sending out — a "self-imposed modesty," says Schneider — and those messages are generally acknowledged with respect. Even today, many authorities "view hair-covering as a part of a married woman's general expression of *tzniut* or personal modesty, a concept which denotes both a physical sense of privacy about one's body as well as a generally inner-directed spiritual quality of personality."[12]

The wearing of the skull cap, or *kippah*, by Jewish males in Orthodox synagogues appears to have been a symbol of just that, being a Jewish male. The rules for modesty and covering one's hair were for women only and coincided with the notion that women are completely responsible for what goes on in the minds of men. (The idea of modesty for Jewish women has, of course, since become a feminist issue.)[13]

There are few allusions to the covering of women's hair in the Torah (the first five books of the Hebrew bible). One is the reference (Gen. 24:65) that Rebekah "took her veil and covered herself"[14] when she first met Isaac (believed to be the act that led to the bride wearing a wedding veil.)[15] Another biblical allusion to hair-covering "occurs in the case of the adulteress, where the High Priest uncovers the head of the woman as a sign of her degradation" — which, according to Schneider, is the basis for the practice of head covering. Hence, it is believed that the tradition of covering women's hair is less a matter of religious doctrine and more a matter of Jewish custom and societal values.[16]

THE VEILING OF MUSLIM WOMEN

In some parts of the world powerful governments reign, making it difficult to understand certain, supposedly religious practices — especially the ones regarding women's dress — and to know if these requirements are indeed theological or political. For example, there is a law in parts of the Middle East — one admonished strongly to be religious — that requires women to be veiled (actually enshrouded) from head to toe; including, of course, the covering of women's hair. Jan Goodwin writes that because religion and state are believed to be one in this part of the world, "leading theologians can wield as much — sometimes more — power than political leaders,"[17] making it difficult for us in the West to understand the stern rulings about women's bodies.

We (in the West) tend to make a common mistake, however, by not differentiating between Middle Eastern culture and Islamic culture. Martha Lee, a young American woman who has converted to the Muslim faith, tells us that most Muslim women do not live in the Middle East:

> India, Pakistan, and Bangladesh are Muslim countries, and India has a significant Muslim population. The former Soviet Republic and China both have Muslim populations of more than sixty million. Malaysia and Indonesia are both Muslim countries; Indonesia is actually the country with the largest Muslim population — around 250 million. Muslims are the second largest religious group in France, and the Muslim population in America is at about six million. The Islamic world is not limited to the Middle East.[18]

For the purposes of this writing, I will explore the covering of Muslim women's hair primarily from a religious position, a view that is based on the Koran, the sacred book of Islam, writings said to be revelations given to Mohammed, the founder of the Muslim religion, by Allah (their god). Whether the law about veiling is religious, cultural, or political, I will leave to the reader.

I am mainly interested in why Muslim women wear the *khimar* — a scarf that covers a woman's hair. Some Muslim women wear the *hijab* — a word that means curtain, or covering, and is a veil that covers the face. [The word curtain is used in the Koran as part of an instruction to followers of Muhammad (in his day) as to how they should deal with his wives.][19] Covering the face, however, is not an obligation for Muslim women, and the majority of Muslim women do not cover their faces. Wearing the khimar, however, is "part of our religion," said Martha. "The way the scarf manifests itself in different cultures is influenced by that culture. But the source of the edict to wear the scarf is from God."

One verse (XXXIII:59) in the Koran that refers to covering the hair (and body), reads: "O Prophet! say to your wives and your daughters, and the women of the believers that they let down upon them their overgarments; this will be more proper, that they may be known, and thus they will not be given trouble,"[20] indicating that covering is for the protection of women. Another verse (XXIV:30) appears to employ covering as a promotion of modesty:

> Enjoin believing women to turn their eyes away from temptation and to preserve their chastity; not to display their adornments (except such as are normally revealed); to draw their veils over their bosoms and not to display their finery except to their husbands, their fathers, their husbands' fathers, their sons, their step-sons, their brothers, their brothers' sons, their sisters' sons, their women-servants and their slave-girls; male attendants lacking in natural vigour, and children who have no carnal knowledge of women.[21]

This may be the verse (or proclamation) that many Muslim women, such as Martha Lee, adhere to. Martha shared that when she dresses for work each morning she doesn't spend time on her hair, her make-up, or worry about which outfit to wear. She is a devoted member of the Muslim faith and has taken herself "out of the competition" — the competition that many women feel as they groom themselves for work each day. Wearing a special outfit, applying make-up, and arranging her hair in a stylish manner is saved for her husband, her family, and her close friends.

Martha Lee has a choice about such matters. She can choose to wear the scarf and throw away the hijab. She lives in America. The law about Muslim women covering their hair (and bodies), however, is said to be interpreted "with varying degrees of strictness from one country to another,"[22] particularly in the Middle East. And wherever the ruling is unheld, it is done so with vehemence. The law is so strict in Tehran that, according to one researcher, signs can be found inside the passenger door of taxis, in stores, restaurants, and in public buildings, a sign that says covering is mandatory. In some areas, storekeepers are forbidden to serve women not covering their hair.[23] Goodwin says,

> The list of violations women can commit in Iran just by dress-ing is long: makeup, nailpolish, and hair showing under the head scarf are just a few. According to Rafsanjani, a man frequently labeled in the West as moderate, "It is the obliga-tion of the female to cover her head because women's hair exudes vibrations that arouse, mislead, and corrupt men."[24]

This is, however, Middle Eastern culture, not Islamic culture. "They are not the same," said Martha. "We as Muslims strive to separate the un-Islamic from the Islamic; we strive to educate our-selves so that we can peel back the layers of culture that have been wrongly attached to our religion." She reminds us that "Middle East-ern culture is misogynistic and overly concerned with sexual honor." She added:

> Yes, a lot of Muslim women cover their hair because it's part of their culture, and they don't dare defy custom. But just as many if not more Muslim women [in other parts of the world] choose to put on the scarf. I've personally known several women who have come from overseas, and when they first come, joyfully abandon wearing the veil. Yet, in a matter of a few months or few years, these same women make the choice to put it back on. And there are women like me who convert to Islam and willingly embrace wearing the veil.

According to one theorist, the shrouding of women's hair (and bodies) was never a law of Mohammed: "fourteen hundred years ago, when Islam began, the Prophet Mohammed permitted women to be politically active, to work and mix with men, and they were not required to veil their faces."[25] Surprisingly, Mohammed is reported to have been among the world's greatest supporters of women's free-dom. Goodwin says,

He abolished such sex-discriminating practices as female in-
fanticide, slavery, and levirate (marriage between a man and
his brother's widow), while introducing concepts guaranteeing
women the right to inherit and bequeath property, and the right
to exercise full possession and control over their own wealth.
Islam, in fact, may be the only religion that formally specified
women's rights and sought ways to protect them.[26]

Yet, one must ponder the knowledge that although Islam (a word
meaning "submission and obedience to the will of God") is intended
to be practiced by all Muslims, only the women are required to dress
themselves to such an extreme. Is it possible, then, that the covering
of women's hair (and bodies) is an attempt to keep them in submission to men?[27]

Western women frequently ask why Islamic women put up with
such strict regulations. Fear, of course, might be one reason — fear
of punishment — especially in Middle Eastern culture. However,
there are other reasons:

1. Covering one's hair is a sign of unification in the church of
   Islam; a symbol of religious sisterhood; a shared female experience.[28]

2. Since Islamic men are probably not going to be tempted by
   shrouded women, the men are less likely to go astray. If all
   women are covered, "wives could rest assured that their hus-
   bands, when not at home, would not encounter a lewd woman
   who might draw his attention away,"[29] reasoned the Iranian
   cleric, Ibrahim Amini.

3. Some women believe that their religion requires them to dress
   modestly, but others say that a more aggressive world moti-
   vates them to cover. Geraldine Brooks supports this theory,
   saying that many Muslim women insist on "going beyond a
   covered head to gloved hands and veiled faces, arguing that
   the corruption of the modern world made more extreme measures necessary now than in the prophet's day."[30] (This doesn't
   mean, however, that Islamic men live at the foot of the cross.
   Bottom-fondling and sexual comments are a problem for
   women, "especially in crowded quarters," writes Brooks, and

"for women in Western dress.")[31]

4. For some it is simply a matter of religion, says Brooks. An Egyptian woman's response to why she covers: "Islam is the answer."[32]

5. The veil is a "useful symbol of respectability among strangers," said Brooks, and a "most effective 'hat' against the merciless sun."[33]

6. Veiling can enhance a woman's mystery and project a vision of willowy grace.[34]

In spite of the seemingly positive reasons why women prefer veiling, there is an apparent controversy (in the East) over the covering of women: where the law originated, what it means, and why it continues. According to one source, it is not a religious custom, never has been, and is simply the outcome of an Islamic extremist movement, patriarchal in nature, and far more political. But since the political behavior of an Islamic force is tightly (and rigidly) bound to religious thought, one can hardly separate the two. Suzanne Campbell-Jones says that

> this is particularly true where Muslim women are concerned. The severe restrictions placed on women by the Islamist movement, such as confinement or complete veiling, have no basis in the Koran or the teachings of the Prophet, but are being stressed because of the role women play in the Muslim world. The honor of the Muslim family is believed to reside in women's chastity and modesty; hence the stress on her being a virgin until her marriage and the very real threat of death if she is not. It is for this reason that the Islamists insist women be completely covered and secluded from the outside world.[35]

THE VEIL OF CATHOLICISM

The Catholic religion is filled with many "things": medals, holy cards, statues, novenas, rosaries, scapulas, famous paintings, and much more. Many of the items are visually appealing — and generally carry an image of Christ, the Blessed Mother, a member of the Holy Family, or a saint. They depict ancient times when men wore beards and mustaches and women had long, straight hair. Monks are depicted with shaved heads (a symbol acknowledging their service to God).[36] Almost all of the women have their hair covered with a veil.

I never gave the idea of holy women and veiling much thought until a few years ago when I was looking through a book about saints and found a photograph of a painting of Mary Magdalene. The painting, by Titian (1477-1576), illustrates a pleasingly plump female, nude from the waist up, with a generous amount of flowing hair, partially covering her breasts. Hence, a woman with a doubtful reputation — Mary Magdalene — is shown with voluptuous, uncovered hair.[37] Her hair was used as a sign of something sexual, no doubt.

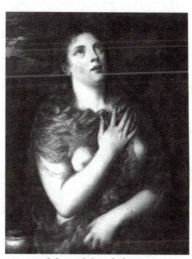

Mary Magdalene

At the opposite end of the hair continuum is a painting of Saint Catherine of Siena dedicating herself to the religious life of chastity or perpetual virginity. In this illustration, Saint Catherine is cutting off her lovely, long hair, while her stern-faced superior sits in observance.[38]

The message is clear, and it supports all of the previously discussed symbolism about hair. If a young woman is dedicating herself and her life to Christ, she must (1) hide an alluring part of her body (that is generally visible and captivating to men), (2) renounce her physical body (neither enhance her appearance nor create an identity), and (3) be dead to the outside world (hair being symbolic of the "life force").

Marcel Bernstein agrees that the ceremonial cutting (or shaving) of women's hair when entering the religious life has its roots in the idea that they [the nuns] "are dying to the world" (a kind of social death) and must reject all that is human, natural, and instinctive. In other words, in a eunuch-type atmosphere one could be successful in dedicating herself to God. She wrote,

A sister who could eradicate her sexuality stood a better chance of becoming holy, and so it became, says an American, "a point of virtue to make oneself unattractive, for attractiveness was a sexual lure." For this reason mirrors were barred, curves were flattened, and heads were shaved — all in the name of virtue.[39]

The Catholic tradition of nuns cutting their hair close to the scalp therefore symbolized the restrained nature of the chastity vow and hiding of all sensuality.[40] And how did these young women feel about having their hair cut off? Some of them embraced their baldness as a "meaningful sacrifice," viewing their clipped heads as a way of being closer to God. Bernstein reports one of the nuns saying, "I can't tell you what immense joy it gave me, being in that condition [having a shaved head]. I'd done it for Him, and this gift of one's hair was something very special." Some of the novices didn't want to be bothered with feminine chores that got in the way of their religious intentions, and they didn't feel that losing their hair was traumatic or problematic. One former nun wrote, "My hair had always been short, and at that point I couldn't wait to wear the headpiece of the habit. Anyway, there wasn't a mirror so I couldn't see how I looked."[41]

Others, however, reported feelings of numbness and dread as the day of the hair-cutting ritual approached. For some, there was a sense of denial about the whole experience. As Mary Gilligan Wong wrote in her memoir about the day she took her temporary vows, "I will do it, then, without thinking, in one fell swoop: I will bow to the scissors that will hack away my long hair, the Rule that will hack away all that is individual, selfish, spontaneous."[42]

Wong said that some of the postulants wept softly as they waited their turn, "watching in dismay" as huge chunks of hair were "chopped off and thrown to the floor." About her own personal experience, she added, "I am stoic as the scissors whack away at my hair with no attention to evenness or style, but when I reach back and feel how jagged it is, how ugly it must look, panic suddenly shoots through the numbness."[43]

In some orders (or novitiates) the hair-cutting ritual took place at random, rather than during the ceremonial reception into the order. Several days after taking her first vows, Midge Turk (formerly Sister Agnes Marie, I.S.M.) was called to the office of her Mother Superior. On the way she passed a tearful friend. Innocently, she entered the office, believing that the meeting was about refitting (or altering) her new habit. Instead, the Reverend Mother was standing next to a straightbacked chair, wearing an apron and holding a set of electric hair clippers. She asked the newly veiled sister to remove her headgear. Midge wrote, "As the long locks fell into my lap I confusedly caught one and kept it clutched in my fist. I had not realized that the shaving of heads was a regulation of the I.H.M. [Immaculate Heart of Mary] community. I had assumed that hair simply would be bobbed."[44]

The full shock of this experience did not get to her until that evening, at bedtime, when she looked into the mirror. "Stunned," she said, "I quickly put on a night coif of soft material that was provided for the purpose." She and two other new novices, in the privacy of the bathroom, tried to comfort one another. She wrote, "In all the years I spent as a religious I never got used to the fact of being without my hair; when uncoiffed I simply avoided looking into mirrors unless it was absolutely necessary." She explained some of the feelings best when she said that losing one's hair was simply a part of the submissive life:

As appalling as shaved heads and spiked arm bands may seem to me now, and did seem to me at the beginning of my novitiate, such things were supported by the unquestioned tradition of formal religious life. In their rightful context, they served a serious purpose and seemed no more horrifying than, say, a circumcision rite for teen-age girls as practiced in the prescribed customs of certain primitive tribes.[45]

Catholicism is not the only religion that requires the cutting (or shaving) of hair when entering the monastic life. Haircutting, sometimes head shaving, is a common tradition among the Buddhists, sometimes simply as a religious practice. Tsultrim Allione says,

Cutting off the hair is done when one renounces the world. Even if monastic vows are not taken, often people going into retreat shave their heads to avoid the time it takes to take care of one's hair and symbolizing the renunciation of vanity. Even when one takes refuge the lama cuts off a strand of hair symbolizing renunciation and creating a bond with the disciple. Hair cutting also symbolizes a new spiritual orientation.[46]

Only one of the women I spoke with, Selena, addressed religious beliefs about her hair.

I grew up in a family that was religious . . . that believed that a woman's hair was supposed to be her glory . . . and should never cut her hair. So, of course, I felt like if I told my mother [that I was experiencing hair loss] it would worry her to death. And, she's my best friend, and I tell her everything. But then, I didn't tell her that. Because I felt that it would really worry her.

IT IS A GLORY TO HER . . .

The idea of a woman's hair being her glory comes from the New Testament (First Corinthians), and reads as follows: "Judge for yourselves; is it proper for a woman to pray to God with her head uncovered? Doth not nature itself teach you that for a man to wear long hair is degrading to him, but if a woman has long hair, it is her pride? For her hair is given to her for a covering.[47]

According to some experts, the passages in this section of the New Testament have less to do with a woman's hair being her honor and glory and more to do with who is whose head, meaning authority, or the "one to whom obedience is due."[48] Further passages read:

But I want you to understand that the head of every man is Christ; and the head of a woman is her husband, and the head of Christ is God. Any man who prays or prophesies with his head covered dishonors his head, but any woman who prays or prophesies with her head unveiled dishonors her head — it is the same as if her head were shaven. For if a woman will not veil herself, then she should cut off her hair; but if it is disgraceful for a woman to be shorn or shaven, let her wear a veil. For a man ought not to cover his head, since he is the image and glory of God; but woman is the glory of man. For man was not made from woman, but woman from man. Neither was man created for woman; but woman for man.[49]

This writing has everything to do with the hierarchical system that existed at that time, and according to Clarence Craig, should be interpreted as follows:

> A Christian man is part of the body of Christ, and Christ is "the head of the body" (Eph. 1:22; 4:15, 5:23; Col. 1:18). That a wife was subordinate to her husband was a teaching of the law (Gen. 3:16) which Paul did not look upon as abrogated in Christ. The subordination of Christ to God is continually affirmed in this letter (3:23; 15:28). In the order of creation each is the head of the one below: God, Christ, man and woman.[50]

This relationship of woman to man is further clarified by Craig as meaning a wife to her husband. Hence, according to Paul, a woman being veiled during a religious service meant that she was inferior to him.[51] Why did men not cover their heads during church services? According to Gundry, it had everything to do with tradition and the "recognition of divinity."[52] And, as stated above, it was about men having authority over women.

There is yet one other interpretation of this biblical verse. Derrett, a professor at the School of Oriental & African Studies (University of London), says the real reason why women were required to cover their hair was its "universal acceptance as a sign of sexual attractiveness." He said that respect had something to do with the head being covered, but primarily "it was the long tresses that needed to be covered." He says the biblical passage should be interpreted as follows: "If a man prays or prophesies with his head covered he treats his head with dishonour.

Whereas if a woman prays or prophesies with her head uncovered she dishonours her head [i.e. her husband!]." Derrett draws on the custom of Jewish women covering their hair while in public, and points out that should she appear bareheaded, "the person injured was her husband."[53]

The biblical notion of man being higher than woman, and the interpretation endorsed by women covering their hair is a practice observed by many religious groups, one such group being the Mennonites. Paul Toews says,

In the MC [Mennonite Church] and various other conserva-
tive Mennonite groups, a crucial symbol for acknowledging
women's submission was the devotional head covering. During the 1920s MC publications ran many articles to advocate
and explain it, almost always based on the apostle Paul's
advice in 1 Corinthians 11:3-10.[54]

An affirmation of this explanation is that during the 1930s there
was concern among the elders of the Mennonite Church that some of
the women (early feminists?) were "usurping man's position and
power" and were scorning their "God-given position of motherhood."
These women were apparently rebelling (by leaving their little white
caps at home).[55]

SAMSON

It seems that most (if not all) biblical male heroes are characterized with an unusual amount of hair, mostly on the head and face.
One of the more famous of these hairy heroes is Samson, a man who
was known for his unusual physical strength and for being a fierce
warrior. Samson was a large man who seemed to be invincible, as he
could survive unbelievable odds. He was so admired for his superior
strength and charisma that he eventually became the leader of the
Israelites and led them in the war against the Philistines. Samson's
weakness, however, was beautiful women. Delilah — a sensual, seductive, and willing female — was the beautiful woman that overcame him and brought about his downfall.[56]
Delilah was bribed by the Philistines to learn the secret of
Samson's phenomenal strength. After much coercing and many tricks,
Delilah was successful. In a moment of great passion, Samson told
Delilah that the secret of his great strength lay in his splendid head
of hair. This, of course, leads to the famous haircut, organized by
Delilah, which robbed Samson of his great physical strength (until
his hair grew back).[57]
It seems that the real message here is not so much about hair
symbolizing physical strength as its representing survival. Samson's
hair symbolizes all of the phenomenal energy that is all about saving
the lives of his people, protecting their land and their lineage (the

life force). Regardless, Gastor says that it is now a "widespread belief that warriors must let their hair grow long lest they loose their strength and invite defeat."[58]

Spiritual Symbolism and the Use of Hair in Ritual

When rituals are conducted within spiritual or religious groups, certain objects are used for symbolic purposes as part of these ceremonies. A frequently used object (for symbolism) in such ceremonies is the cranial hair. E. R. Leach, a well-known anthropologist, says that hair represents "some kind of metaphysical abstraction — fertility, soul-stuff, personal power."[59] Theodore Gastor says that it is used symbolically as a "life-index," or as the "seat of the vital spirit" (and "may not be cut during the first year of life lest future health and vigor be impaired.")[60] There are various explanations about what hair means in these activities, but there is one overall spiritual meaning that persists. Because hair can regenerate itself, it has become a symbol of life and the life force — that unseen energy that propels us forward on our journey through life.[61]

In certain cultures, the first haircut takes place during a religious ceremony. For example, when children belonging to one of the Toradjas tribes[62] had their hair cut, a portion was always left on the crown, the belief being that if all of the hair was cut, the soul would be deprived of a place to live and the child would become ill. In similar tribes, this patch of hair remained uncut all through life, or at least until manhood.[63]

Hair has received similar respect in the Siamese culture. J. G. Frazier says that

> when the topknot of a Siamese child has been cut with great ceremony, the short hairs are put into a little vessel made of plantain leaves and set adrift on the nearest river or canal. As they float away, all that was wrong or harmful in the child's disposition is believed to depart with them. The long hairs are kept till the child makes a pilgrimage to the holy Footprint of Buddha on the sacred hill at Prabat. They are then presented to the priests, who

are supposed to make them into brushes with which they sweep the Footprint.[64]

Among the Hos, a tribe of West Africa, there are priests who believe that head hair is "the seat and lodging place" of their god, "so that were it shorn the god would lose his abode in the priest." For this reason some of the priests live their entire lives without cutting their hair; the belief being that "the god who dwells in the man forbids the cutting of his hair on pain of death."[65] In this case the head hair seems to represent a connection with spiritual strength or a source of everlasting life.

In certain primitive cultures in the South Pacific, cutting the hair or shaving the head was a way of giving something to the gods, an offering to ward off evil influences. For example, on some of the Fiji Islands, a bride might offer a lock of hair to the gods. In some cases her head was completely shaved.[66] Gastor says that in surrendering the hair, one is surrendering his or her "essential *life-spirit*," an appropriate gesture whenever an individual "assumes a new character," such as becoming a wife. "It was a common practice in antiquity to shear one's locks and dedicate them to the deity at the moment one reached puberty and 'put away childish things.'"[67] (This may explain why, in some parts of the world, it was common to cut the hair of a Jewish boy on or about his thirteenth birthday — at the time of his *bar mitzvah*, or coming of age.)[68]

The practice of cutting the hair of a new bride is apparently quite common. According to Gastor,

> In ancient Greece, the bride's tresses were cut before marriage and dedicated to the goddess; while among the Romans they were parted with the so-called "bachelor's spear" before the nuptial ceremony. In the steppes of Southeast Russia, on the shores of the Caspian and Black Seas, the bride has her hair cut off when she returns home after visiting relatives and friends on the eve of her wedding.[69]

In other areas of the world the head itself is regarded as sacred; it is believed to contain a spirit, says Frazier, "which is very sensitive to injury or disrespect." The Siamese, Cambodians, and Polynesians believe that a "guardian spirit" (the *kuan* or *kwun*) dwells in the human head and that the head must never be touched by a stranger. Consequently, great care is taken with the cranial hair, and hair care "is accompanied with many ceremonies." In these cultures hair-cutting especially is a delicate procedure — and particularly distressing for the hairdresser who is afraid of disrupting the spirit.[70] According to Richard Corson, this practice began in ancient civilizations:

> Since it was believed among many superstitious peoples that the guardian spirit of the head might be injured or inconvenienced, the hair was not frequently washed, and when it was, the occasion often became a ceremonial one, especially among royalty. According to Herodotus, the head of the king of Persia was washed only on his birthday.[71]

Such superstitions about the hair persisted through ancient Roman times, said Corson. Roman women only washed their hair once a year, "on the birthday of Diana, the thirteenth of August."[72]

The fact that the cranial hair grows out of the head — the seat of mindful activities — there may be a logical explanation for the hair-soul-God connection. However, "the link between hair and spiritual and magical power is slightly more complex."[73]

THE SYMBOLIC USE OF HAIR IN WITCHCRAFT, MAGIC, AND DEVIL-LORE

A. S. Gregor writes that "rituals are the magical means by which men try to make their wishes come true," with two categories of magic described: imitative and contagious. Imitative magic is based on the belief that items resembling one another "affect each other" (i.e., sticking pins in an image, like a doll, that resembles one's victim). The theory in contagious magic is that "things once in contact remain in such a close relationship that what is done to one is done to the other."[74] Hair is used frequently in both types of magic.

A good example of how hair is used in imitative magic is offered in Kittredge's work on witchcraft. He reports that in 1594, an image (made of wax) of Ferdinando, the fifth Earl of Derby, was found in his bedroom with a hair "prict directly in the heart." The earl had died suddenly, and foul play was suspected as the hair belonged to an old woman.[75] In imitative magic, hair is not always used for evil intent, however. Sometimes it is used in ritual cures for the sick, whereby hair combings of living enemies of the patient — who are believed to be the cause of the illness — are bound with imitative statues and buried in the ground.[76]

Because a lock or strand of hair is believed to remain connected to its former owner (contagious magic), hair has been and still is used for magical purposes. In East Africa, guards did not have to stand over a prisoner. Gregor says that "if a few locks were cut from his hair he dared not escape." In keeping with that a relationship exists with the hair even after it has been cut — and that whatever happens to the loose hair (which could be desecration), happens to the owner.[78] Corson said that

> the Egyptian custom of letting the hair grow when away from one's own country apparently was grounded not so much in a desire to conform to foreign customs as to avoid possible dangers arising from unfamiliar and presumably evil spirits who might get at one in a foreign land through clippings of the hair.[79]

Similar practices are also used in problems with romance. Gregor relates a story whereby a young Native American, from a tribe known as the Blackfeet, fell in love with a maiden "who rejected all his advances until one day he stole a lock of her hair." The Indian maiden "fell under his power and followed him both day and night" until, overwhelmed and harassed, he finally returned her hair.[77]

P. Bohannon reports that an Italian (to this day) may not give a lock of hair to anyone "lest he should be bewitched or enamoured against his will"[80] (meaning that should it fall into the wrong hands, his or her life could be in danger). For this reason, in some parts of the world, cut hair is carefully preserved in order to be protected from a sorcerer, particularly in the Malay Peninsula.[81]

On the other hand, the hair of a witch was believed to protect her powers. Cooper says that in years past, in both Europe and India the head of a suspected witch was shaved, and in some cases the whole body was shaved — "partly to search for hidden marks of Satanic allegiance, and partly to deprive her of the strength and protection she derived from her hair."[82] W. Crooke tells us that, in Bastar (a village in northern India), if a man was found practicing witchcraft, his hair was shaved, the substance believed "to constitute his power of mischief."[83]

According to Moncure Conway, the fact that hair is a powerful, magical, and sometimes demonic substance is believed to have originated from the legend of Lilith, Adam's first wife in Jewish legend — a female who supposedly had potent tresses and "was a first wife that turned out badly."[84] As the legend goes, Lilith was not created from Adam's rib, but was created at the same time as Adam — setting up an argument about who was in charge — and Adam wouldn't back down. Lilith became so angry about the inequality in her relationship with Adam that she uttered a spell, the result being that she "obtained wings" and flew away.[85] Lilith and Adam eventually divorced, leaving Lilith to grieve over the loss of Eden and enticing her into some rather evil activities; one being that she took the form of a serpent and was allegedly responsible for the temptation of Eve.[86]

And this is where her fatal locks come in. The arts portray Lilith as more beautiful than Eve — and with long, flowing hair. Michaelangelo's painting of Lilith on the ceiling of the Sistine Chapel illustrates her as "a marvellous [sic] beauty." And Rossetti, a poet of the nineteenth century, depicts Lilith as "the mediaeval witch against whose beautiful locks Mephistopheles warns Faust when she appears at the Walpurgis-night orgie."

> The rose and poppy are her flowers; for where
> Is he not found, O Lilith, whom shed scent
> And soft-shed kisses and soft sleep shall snare?
> Lo! as that youth's eyes burned at thine, so went
> Thy spell through him, and left his straight neck bent,
> And round his heart one strangling golden hair.[87]

In many art forms, there is a warning against a beautiful woman with fatal locks, and Lilith appears to be the first of this long line of generously tressed seductresses. Is it possible, then, that the words of Paul — saying that a woman's hair is her glory — suggest that hair has a prior, ominous reputation? "Such glory might easily be degraded," writes Conway, "and every hair turn to a fatal 'binder,' like the one golden thread of Lilith round the heart of her victim; or it might ensnare its owner."[88] (It is important to note that, according to legend, Eve's long hair was trimmed by God before she was given to Adam.[89])

Head hair has enormous symbolic power in almost every culture, especially within religious circles. The meanings assigned to this part of the body vary from group to group, but generally they are associated with a spiritual being (God or Allah) or an invisible energy (life force), often reflecting magical thinking, with rituals frequently involving a special cutting, covering, and sometimes preserving of hair. On the other hand, a woman's hair has been traditionally viewed as provocative or dangerous (irreligious) — so much so that it has brought about social and religious laws forbidding women to wander about without head coverings. Such laws are still in effect in some parts of the world.

The head coverings of Catholic and Jewish women and holy women in the Bible signify purity, modesty, and goodness. The veil of a Catholic sister symbolizes her marriage to Christ, her virginity, and the hiding of her sexuality. Because a woman's hair represents her sexual nature (according to certain religious beliefs) and because nonmarital sex is a sin (according to certain religious teachings), in some parts of the world, even a lay woman's hair was required to be tamed or hidden. Lay Catholic women covered their hair when in church for a time in history. The Jewish woman's head covering (when outside her home) protected her honor, her marriage, and her family. For a Jewish woman to let her hair hang down and have a disheveled appearance was actually a sign of being shut off from the community, such as being a prostitute or a vamp. It was a sign of having loose morals, and if proven true, her hair was whacked off as a punishment. (By the New Testament era, Jews were no longer permitted to execute women for adultery, and the punishment became the cutting of her hair, along with expulsion from the synagogue.)[90] The small cap worn by the women in the Mennonite church is a badge of submission, an announcement and a reminder of their place in the church hierarchy.

Hair is also a powerful substance within the world of magic, witchcraft and demonology, with its roots traced back to Lilith. Legend tells us that the beautiful Lilith had lovely, long, lethal hair. She was also a troublemaker, hovering outside the garden of Eden. Since that time, the power of witches (and warlocks) is believed to reside in their hair, with strands and locks of hair frequently being used in casting spells.

With all of the power that is assigned to hair, no wonder its loss is so devastating!

CHAPTER FIVE

THE MANE ATTRACTION

The Sensual and Romantic Aspects of Hair

THE COCK OF HIS COMB

Mr. Geddys was frantic. His son, Victor, had disappeared, abandoning his cancer treatment, his care givers, and his familiar and comfortable surroundings. When

> The tresses long about her face — a living censer, left the place, with strange, wild odours all astir. . .
> — Charles Baudelaire

he found Victor in Mendicino County — at a romantic hideaway — he was angry and upset. By now, of course, Victor, too, was distraught — stopping his cancer treatment had caused his symptoms to return; a deception that also resulted in his lover's angry and unforgiving departure. Mr. Geddys asked, "Why did you do this [stop the chemotherapy]? The treatment . . . how could you walk away in the middle of it?" Victor wept and calmly replied, "I wanted her to see me with hair."[1]

In *Dying Young*, a heavyhearted movie about love, life, and loss — Victor sacrificed his life in order to grow his hair; to look attractive (and sexy) to Hillary, the woman he desires.[2] It isn't unusual for people to have such strong feelings about their hair. Hair represents the sensual and sexual qualities of both sexes — the qualities that, no doubt, make it something of a romantic substance. A curl, tied with a dainty ribbon, is sent to a loved one — a sensual offering of the self, perhaps. Soldiers have been known to carry a lock of their beloved's hair into battle — maybe for comfort. A widow might bury a lock with her husband's body.[3] Locks of hair have also been preserved keepsakes of lost loved ones — generally in a locket, pin, or bracelet — the belief being that it can create a sacred connection or union with the dead.[4] These are loving, tender gifts and remembrances that we never give much thought to. Yet we instinctively know that hair is sensual. One romantic wrote:

> I once tucked a perfect curl of my hair, tied with a lavendar ribbon, between the pages of a poetry book I was returning to a friend. The curl marked my favorite love poem, and I felt as if I were charging the book with my life force. I knew I was giving him a powerful talisman. Hair is sacred to lovers . . .[5]

Hair is frequently mentioned in love songs and poems. "Here, There, and Everywhere," a famous melody by John Lennon and Paul McCartney, flows with loving, sensual lyrics — one, in particular, alluding to running one's hands through the lover's hair.[6] In a well-known work by Lord Byron, *Maid of Athens, ere we part*, the lover's hair is poetically versed as "unconfined tresses" blowing in the wind.[7] While in another, he woos "every raven tress" of the beloved.[8]

"Yielding and soft, sumptuous and dangling," hair invites a lover's touch, said Ackerman.[9] There is more to this lover's phenomenon, however, than just sight and touch. The sight, touch and smell of hair — most of our senses — seem to enter into our relationship with hair.

THE SENSUAL ASPECTS OF HAIR

We have already discussed the theory that hair was important to our ancestors when looking for a mate. If you recall, the male with the most impressive hair frightened away his rivals, winning the female of his choice. Females with long, healthy hair — believed to represent good health (for childbearing) — were prized in coupling. Even today, hair — as part of one's sexual appeal and physical attractiveness — is important to us when looking for a partner.

As mentioned in Chapter Three, hair is believed to be sexual on a subconscious level, a theory strongly supported (perhaps unknowingly) by certain religious groups. There are even more theories associated with hair — sexual in nature — that may help us understand why we have romantic and sensual feelings about this part of the body. The first is related to puberty, the time in life when we are becoming sexual beings and beaming with signs of this physical, mental and emotional change. The second is related to another, less obvious part of our biological and psychological nature: Odors (pheromones) that are secreted through hairy parts of the body, including the scalp, and that lure us subconsciously into flirtations and sexual encounters.

When one enters puberty, there is excess growth of hair all over the body. For women, hair appears under the arms, in the pubic area, and sometimes around the nipples. For men, the growth is more pervasive: on the face, chest, axillary and pubic regions, and simply all over the body. This secondary growth of hair announces the physical readiness to be sexually active. It is a sign of sexual maturity and a symbol of virility and fertility. In various cultures, this same role is given "with no real biological justification" to the hair on the head.[10] In other words, hair growth coinciding with puberty, may be partly responsible for our sexual fascination with the scalp hair. Because men grow so much hair as they develop sexually, it becomes the badge of manhood — an emblem of virility. Perhaps one reason why men do not want to lose their hair.

Several of the men I spoke with indicated that this may indeed be so. Bruce, who was going through a marital separation, spoke of his concerns about dating again. He said he was afraid he might be rejected because of his hair loss: "It's unlikely that I will be picking up a lady friend at a bar next week. But, if I were to get shot down or rejected because of this . . . just the thought in my head is enough to get me distressed." He acknowledged that his hair loss had sometimes been an issue in his failing marriage. "You know, if you're not confident in yourself in terms of your looks, your sexuality. It can be a big downer."

When discussing changes in his life after he lost his hair, Thomas said, "I think that I'm maybe less attractive to the opposite sex." He said that he was told repeatedly by women that they were either attracted to bald men or that it didn't matter to them at all. "But that still doesn't put out of my mind the possibility that it might be something that's not appealing to someone else. I think the problem is more mine than it is the other person's. I don't feel like I'm as attractive to the ladies as I would be with more hair."

Mark, who is experiencing male pattern baldness, said that he had never had any problems meeting girls and getting dates, but now he notices what he doesn't have. He said that if he overhears a girl saying, "Oh, there's a guy who's really good looking," he says to himself, "If only I had a full head of hair that I could do something with, like the total stud-looking guy." And Don said, "If I go into an environment where there's one hundred men and no women around, I feel pretty confident. I've always — for whatever reason — felt pretty socially successful in that way." But that wasn't his big concern.

> I don't much care what guys think. And if I'm in a relationship, then I don't pretty much care what anybody else thinks. I kinda care what the person I'm with thinks. When I wasn't in a relationship, yeah, it bothered me a lot more. Because then you think it's kind of preemptive.

Another man that I spoke with said,

> At my age, a big thing is sex appeal. To my wife, to others ... I want to be sexually appealing. I work very hard to keep in shape at the gym, at the pool, whatever. I am very, very comfortable with my body. But I think, *Wouldn't it be nice to tie in a great hairdo?* So that is emotionally very hard for me, that it doesn't matter how my body looks, I'll always be uncomfortable with my hair. If my appearance does not give me the confidence to be comfortable around women that I find appealing. You know, 'Boy, he's a nice guy. He's got a nice body and everything. But shit! He's bald!'

Roger said that when he left home to attend a state university he was feeling somewhat frustrated with his physical appearance, mainly because he was already losing hair. He said that he wanted to "look more normal." He wanted to be dating, and he wanted young women to be attracted to his appearance. So he started using Rogaine brand of minoxidil and began to regain his nice head of hair. He was feeling pretty good about himself, and this is when his relationship with Carol began.

Then Roger began to experience some negative side effects from the medication. He had to stop using Rogaine; six months later he was back to experiencing hair loss, which was emotionally distressing. He said that one of the good outcomes, however, was the response that he got from Carol: She was "very open-minded about it, very understanding, very supportive."

In the early stages of the relationship, Roger said he asked himself, "What if I had not found Rogaine? Would she [Carol] have seen me differently? Would I have had the confidence to ask her out?" He didn't have the answers to those questions, of course. But he said that he probably would have been a lot more concerned about his appearance, "and stressed out about how I looked." Sadly, I received a letter from Roger sometime later telling me that Carol had ended their relationship. He sounded quite depressed about it, and told me that his hair loss was once again causing him to feel less attractive to the opposite sex. Consequently, he was once again worried about dating.

Don may have captured Roger's feelings when he said,

> I think younger people in both genders are looking for a trophy. And being bald, you're probably not going to fit into the trophy category as much. Any woman who is with me, I'm always gonna have this one particular kind of non-trophylike status. I would imagine it's not altogether different than a woman who doesn't have any breasts or something else along those lines.

Bret may have shed some light on this too, when he expressed the feeling that "baldness equals some sort of inadequacy or less desirability."

Hair Loss in Women and the Loss of Sexual-Esteem

Balding causes some men to feel less attractive to the opposite sex. Women, however, feel considerably less attractive and undesirable if they lose their hair. In writing about her experience with total hair loss, Jojuan J. Lamorreaia said that she finally did begin wearing wigs and that she eventually resumed a functional lifestyle — but she always expected rejection when she broke the news to a potential partner that she had no hair.[11]

The men that I spoke with feared rejection, but the women expected it. Sheila said she knew that once a man found out that she didn't have any hair, it would change things, so she doesn't let a potential mate get very close. Melissa said, "It's hard for me with meeting guys. It's hard for me to approach a guy." She added, "These days, you know, they just stand around and wait for you to come to them. That's kind of hard for me to do. I think they may realize that I'm wearing a wig."

Yolanda said that her hair loss had made her feel less feminine: "... less than a woman. When you lose your ability to feel comfortable sexually with somebody, a major part of who you are, and a major part of your emotions become restricted." Yolanda did not begin to look for a new partner until her hair was growing back in. Hattie didn't even want her husband to know. "He didn't know anything about it 'cause I was trying to keep it from him, 'cause I didn't know how he was gonna accept that." She added, "Who wants a baldheaded woman?"

All of the individuals I spoke with — both men and women — used many of the same words to describe the emotional experience of losing their hair. Women, however, expressed greater emotional distress than men. This is not a shocking revelation, given that women often feel pressured to define themselves through their appearance, especially the sensual or sexual self. How a woman views her body and physical attractiveness is closely connected with self-worth, and distortion of one can distort the other. So, if a woman fails to retain her attractiveness — as would happen with hair loss — she begins to feel helpless with controlling one of the fundamental aspects of her feminine identity.[12] "Our hair, after all, is not a vain, superficial obsession but a mythic symbol of power — Samson's downfall, Rapunzel's salvation, Lorelei's seductive, blinding tool — and a quirky, spiritual barometer of precisely what's most meaningful for us,"[13] says Dalma Heyn.

A woman's need to hide the fact that she is balding reflects an already pervasive problem that women face in our society — that of having to be different (and more) than who they really are. Women are not given the message that their bodies are valuable "simply because they are inside them," wrote Naomi Wolf. Instead they are given the message that they must above all be physically attractive and that they must have all of their physical parts.[14] Selena said,

> You know. It's being women. Even though men feel shame, it's an accepted thing that they will lose their hair at a certain point. People know that male pattern baldness is common. But, even though women do lose their hair, it's something we just don't associate with women.

The difference, then, in male and female relationships to their bodies may lie in a basic social phenomenon: Men have power and control in the world just because they are men. A woman's way of competing with this power (and attempting to feel valuable in the world) is generally with her charm and physical appearance.[15] Hence, a woman's lush, long hair can give her a kind of sexual authority in the world. Any woman who has "swung her head around and felt her hair fall seconds afterward like thick velvet ribbons has experienced [this] a taste of power," says Heyn.[16]

As mentioned in an earlier chapter, males, as well as females, are effected by the forces of physical attractiveness: a male image that is portrayed or thrust before humankind; an image that was predominantly blamed on the media. Jake blamed it on the fashion industry: "It's that point zero five percent of our population that just looks amazing."

THE SEDUCTIVE (AND SUBCONSCIOUS) SCENT OF HAIR

There is more to the sexual fascination of hair than presenting a sexy appearance, or fondling and caressing it. In Corbin's work, *The miasme et la jonquille* [*The Foul and the Fragrant*], the scalp hair is identified as one of the seven parts of the body that gives off secretions or odors related to purging or cleansing — natural odors, which are believed to be seductive through their delicate smell.[17] In addition, W. Montagna wrote that large numbers of sebaceous glands are located "on the scalp, forehead, cheeks, and chin," and these glands are controlled by sex hormones.[18] Michael Stoddard, also, identified the scalp as one of the major scent-gland regions of the human body. He identified 17 sites of scent production — all of them with excess hair — and wrote that the "quality of odour produced by human scent glands … links odour production with sexual communication."[19] He said that

> The naso-hypothalamic-hypophysial-gonadal link is as strong in humans as it is in other mammals, even though it may be difficult immediately to accept that our sense of smell plays much of a role in human reproduction. Human males do not react to pheromones in the way that male dogs do for example to the odour of a bitch in heat, but the ancient linkage, however, remains quite intact.[20]

Consistent with the scent-gland [naso-hypothalamic-hypophysial-gonadal] theory, researchers have discovered a sense organ inside the human nose — an organ that is believed to pick up the seductive scent of other humans. This small organ — measured to be a half inch or so in length — is called the vomeronasal organ (VNO). It is believed to detect chemical signals sent unconsciously from one human being to another, such as through the hair on the head. K. Wright said that these hormonal scents (or signals), called pheromones, "might be about identity, arousal, or sexual receptivity."[21]

The scent and smell role in mating behavior among animals has been known for years. But it was believed that human beings were more socialized and civilized and that we were getting things accomplished without resorting to such a primitive system. Apparently the exchange of pheromones among human beings does exist, but, of course, is not detected consciously. Wright said that "unlike conscious sensations [such as touch] the messages conveyed via the VNO would bypass mental awareness and make a beeline for the primitive brain."[22] According to Stoddart, odours seem to speak to the deepest levels of the unconscious mind; those parts of the mind where only great artists are privileged to wander, and from where most of humankind is barred. "Much can be learned from the writings of the philosophers," he wrote, "from introspective creations of writers and artists and from psychoanalysts who probe the unconscious about odour symbolism, and about the special relationship which exists between the nose and the psyche."[23] The odor that they are referring to is musk.[24]

According to Desmond Morris, the attraction that one individual has for another involves liking the way a potential partner smells: "We know that there are sex differences in body odours and it has been suggested that part of the process of pair-formation — falling in love — involves a kind of olfactory imprinting, a fixation on the specific individual odour of the partner's body."[25] He also discusses the particular odors, sexual in nature, to which humans are drawn.

> Before puberty there are strong preferences for sweet and fruity odours, but with the arrival of sexual maturity this response falls off and there is a dramatic shift in favour of flowery, oily and musky odours. This applies to both sexes, but the increase in musk responsiveness is stronger in males than females. It is claimed that as adults we can detect the presence of musk even when it is diluted down to one part in eight million parts of air, and it is significant that this substance plays a dominant role in the scent-signalling of many mammalian species, being produced in specialized scent glands.[26]

For centuries our more colorful writers have alluded to the sexual scent of humans, often with regard to the hair on the head. Havelock Ellis said that because of its smell and touch, hair has been particularly useful as a fetish. Ellis spoke of fondling the hair, and he also spoke of musk — the odor that seems to linger in the hair — as having a particularly sexual odor. And he referred to Firdusi's writings, where Firdusi "speaks of a woman's hair as 'a crown of musk'" — and the offerings of Arabian poet, Motannabi.[27]

In his work, *Poems of Al-Motannabi*, Motannabi writes extensively (and sensually) about his attraction to the hair — or "tresses" — of the young maidens of his youth: how it smelled ("musk"); the color ("pitch black"); the curls, braids, and tangles; the thickness.[28]

Perhaps the most famous poetic writing about hair, however, is "The Rape of the Lock," by Alexander Pope. Based on an actual event, this comical satire reflects the sexual symbolism of hair, along with the shock and outrage that resulted from a young gent, Lord Petre (a suitor), cutting and stealing a lock from a well-known young woman, Miss Arabella Fermor. The incident quickly became a scandal, according to Wendy Cooper, mainly because the Fermor family was outraged that Petre would take such liberties with their daughter. Alexander Pope, who was summoned to "pour poetic oil onto troubled social waters," created an even bigger problem when he didn't take the incident seriously enough. In fact, he poked fun at it.[29]

In this humorous work, the predator (named "Baron") approaches his beloved's hair seductively — in the same manner as he would woo her into his bed.[30] (Hence, the rape of the lock.)

Hair is a romantic, sensual, and sexual symbol that most of us wear proudly and want to present to the world. It is part of love-making — fun to play with while flirting: "Messing it up is the symbolic equivalent of undressing the other's body," wrote Ackerman.[31] Roberta (and one other individual) compared a woman's hair to the female's breasts. She added that it wasn't a matter of "just being sexy for men, it's being sexy for society, for your group. And sexy — maybe it's the wrong term — but it's the gut term. If you really want to get to what is attraction. And, it's the animal word."

Our hair is so important to us, especially on romantic and sexual levels. As demonstrated by the people I spoke with, it is vital for the sexual self-esteem and in wanting to attract and hold a mate, in sensuality, and in appearing adequately masculine or feminine. Almost everyone I spoke with discussed a changed perception of themselves (as balding individuals) in relation to the opposite sex, such as a lack of confidence in dating.

None of the individuals that I spoke with mentioned a "sexual scent" (the release of pheromones that linger in the hair and send a sexual signal to a potential partner), but why would they? This is a subconscious experience that is only recently being recognized by scientists. The discovery, however, does help us unravel the mystery of why and how the head hair plays a role in flirtation and foreplay.

Clearly, women feel a loss of sexual power when they lose their hair. Most of the men that I spoke with revealed that they feel a loss of sexual appeal. For many, it is an emotionally complicated experience that involves far more than concern about body image.

Part II

OVERCOMING THE TRAUMA OF HAIR LOSS

CHAPTER SIX

A PRIVATE AND SILENT MOURNING

Grieving the Loss of One's Hair

THE LOSS OF A PART OF THE SELF

Loss. It comes in many forms — sometimes through choice, now and then through neglect, often through death. Sometimes it's something over which we have no control: a lover or partner wants space, a home is destroyed by natural forces, jobs are eliminated by companies in transition. Sometimes we lose a part of the body. "Loss of a body part," wrote Simos, "can be as devastating as the loss of a significant person"[1] — a breast to cancer, a limb to accident, the eyes to diabetes, hair to unknown causes.

> There are worse things than hair loss, but it's sometimes hard to remember what they are.
> — Renata Polt

The death of a loved one is, of course, the ultimate loss. Death is final and complete. But many little deaths are suffered by all of us along the way. Divorce, desertion, separation, abortion, stillbirth, and rejection mean losses of significant people. Equally as devastating as the loss of a significant person can be the loss of a part of the self ... or any outward change that disrupts body image.[2]

Any significant loss can be a frightening, painful experience. Losing one's hair, however, offers an anguish all of its own. Along with the primary loss of body image, the secondary losses — the social, cultural, and psychological entanglements — that accompany this unwanted change make it a complicated and emotionally troubling ordeal, especially for women.[3]

Mourning the Loss of One's Hair

Jojuan J. Lamorreaia agonized over the loss of her hair. She hid from the world, and tried desperately to find a cure. She was devastated. She became depressed, even suicidal. She sought the help of many doctors, tried various treatments, "even steroids — getting 30 to 40 injections" into her scalp at a time. Sadly, the injections didn't help. They only made her situation worse; she gained about 70 pounds. She finally tried wearing a wig, but nothing released her from the painful fact that she was bald.[4]

Renata Polt lost all of her hair following chemotherapy treatments for cancer. Even though she'd been warned, even told that it would grow back, she was stunned. She said that her hair didn't come back all at once. She remembers dressing one evening to attend a party, and when she ran the comb through her hair, "there it was." She knew that it would happen: chemotherapy kills not only cancer cells but "other fast-growing, fast-dividing cells such as those in hair follicles." But all of the knowledge and preparation didn't help.[5]

However, the shock of losing her hair didn't hit Renata until the next day "when the stuff started coming out in handfuls." It was then that she had her first crying jag — the first of two— since learning that she had breast cancer.[6]

Men do not like to lose their hair — but when a woman loses her hair she is robbed of a valuable asset, an important aspect of her appearance, sexuality, and femininity. As Renata said during our meeting, "I would assume that men grow up knowing that someday they might lose their hair, but for a woman, it is unacceptable!"

What I learned through listening to people with hair loss, however, is that some men — as well as women — truly grieve the loss of their hair. Furthermore, men and women experience this loss in similar ways. Almost all of the individuals that I spoke with used many of the same words to describe their feelings. They didn't like the way that they looked, and this appeared to affect their self-esteem;[7] hair loss inevitably brings a threat to self-esteem.[8] Everyone discussed a changed perception of themselves in relation to the opposite sex (which disturbed them greatly). They spoke openly about the different stages of mourning. Yolanda said, "I lost a part of me. And I didn't want to lose that. So that's painful." Mark, who was 21 years old at the time of our meeting, agreed: "You're in the process of losing your hair. You're losing something! People don't like to lose things, you know?" Bruce said, "You go from a certain way that you liked the way that you looked. It wasn't fun."

When I asked Grace if she remembered the emotional aspect of her hair loss experience, she said, "I certainly do remember. I remember a lot of it — you know, as far as the way I felt." She said:

> I can remember looking at pictures of myself when I was in the hospital. My brother came to visit. Probably two days after I had the stroke he was in North Carolina. And, there's a picture of me sitting in a wheelchair with him, you know ... kind of leaning down hugging me, or something. And I look perfectly normal. I mean, I could not move the entire left side of my body, but I looked okay And now, six months afterwards, when I was supposedly okay, I was looking very ill. And it was like one more thing to have to go through. 'Cause there had been just this series of things, and now I was losing my hair.

Hair loss inflicts a radical change in physical appearance, especially if it happens suddenly and quickly (as with Grace); even a slow process of balding, however, feels drastic and life-altering. Jake said that he hadn't done much in high school, that he hadn't participated much in group activities and hadn't made a lot of friends. Losing his hair was a "huge loss," because he was hoping that college would be something different. The change in his appearance put a damper on his vision of expanding his lifestyle.

Others spoke of losing self-confidence. Yolanda said, "I think it's more than a loss of physical attractiveness. Because for me, it was a loss of confidence. It was a loss of self-confidence." Mark said that, for him, it was definitely a confidence shaker in the beginning, especially in his freshman year in college. "Like, here I am entering adulthood and I've got aspects of adulthood I don't want yet. I know for a while there it was definitely a confidence thing."

A loss of self-confidence in individuals experiencing hair loss may have something to do with social comparison. Individuals generally feel more comfortable when they believe that they look relatively similar to the other people in their environment.[9] They can also feel somewhat uncomfortable, oftentimes inferior, if they are acutely aware of differences — especially differences that are perceived as negative. Jake said that it was tough to lose his hair at such a young age. "It was difficult to sort of feel hampered before you get out of the gate, and be able to have self-confidence, and look like other guys who still have a lot of hair."

Bruce said that he used to feel more sure of himself before he lost his hair:

> I used to be a very, very vocal person; very much a type of leader through high school; through college I was swim team captain, group leader of various projects, tons of self-confidence, just very happy with myself. I was never afraid of saying how I felt. It [hair loss] has changed my life in various ways.

Several of the men said they were viewed as older than they really were — like Jake — and they mourned the loss of their youth (a typical concern in Western society). Don said:

> Sometimes it [being bald] made me feel old. Like my very first day at Carolina. I didn't know anything. And a girl, who was my age — you know, an incoming freshman — came up to me and wanted to ask me directions. And she stopped me, and she said, 'Excuse me, sir.' And I was like, 'WHOA! Wait a second! I'm 18 years old! I'm no sir!'

Mark added, "It's definitely considered the end of the independent life, so to speak. Like, as you're going bald, you're past the peak. Your youth is over, you know? The glory days are gone. The next thing is retirement."

The idea of aging (and being viewed as older) creates a stressful and undesirable life event; one for which young men are not prepared. (Balding men are frequently judged to be about five years older than they really are.[10]) Bret said that being viewed as older was "irritating." He said if he hadn't lost his hair, nobody would have assumed he was any older than they were. He said that people related to him in a different way: " People start calling you sir and not that that's the kiss of death or anything. But you know that to them, there's something different about you from who they are. You know, like college students . . . an older guy in the class."

"There are feelings and stages common to all forms of loss," wrote Ira Tanner, "up to eleven in all: shock, sobbing, craziness, relief, physical symptoms of unresolved grief, panic, guilt, anger, limbo, hope emerges, reality is affirmed."[11] Almost all of the individuals I spoke with were enduring one or more of these stages while mourning the loss of their hair. They talked about denial, shock and alarm during the initial stage. Several spoke of bargaining with God and promising to do certain things if their hair would just grow. Many indicated a feeling of helplessness. Anger was expressed, as was sadness. Several of the women said that they had cried repeatedly over their hair loss. A feeling of guilt was reported — what did I do to cause this? Both men and women spoke of shame, and made efforts to hide their baldness. The feelings of grief were related to losing a body part and body image (the concept we hold in our minds of our bodies),[12] with the greatest concern being a perceived loss of sexual attractiveness. In spite of ongoing hair loss, several of the people that I interviewed appeared to be entering the final stages of mourning when they spoke of acceptance. Their words follow.

Denial, Shock, and Alarm

Walt said, "I think I reacted by trying to pretend like it wasn't happening because it was so moderate. It was so mild at the beginning. I said, 'Well, if I'm losing my hair I'll figure it out in a couple of months, I guess'." Grace said that at first she ignored the fact that her hair was falling out. "Maybe I just completely denied it, you know? Like, this is something that will go away."

The first phase of grieving hair loss — and one of the more recognizable stages — is disbelief in the fact that the loss is occurring.

Denial "serves as a cushion," writes Tanner, "giving us time to absorb the fact of loss. We hear the words of loss [or see the loss], but we do not feel the loss."[13] Jake's comment on when he discovered that his hairline was receding is a perfect example of denial:

> So I was looking at it, and then I noticed that my hair was thinning. There wasn't much there. And I started realizing that, Wow! So I decided to comb my hair to the side instead of parting it down the middle. And the whole morning it was like, "Okay. Okay. You're just feeling a little different. And you're feeling a little outside of yourself." It's just so slight in the beginning, you figure, "Oh, it's just my eyesight. There's nothing to be alarmed about here."

Roger said that initially he, too, was in denial. He remembered a friend saying, "Hey! You're losing your hair." He replied, "Ah, no I don't think so." Mark said that he was forced to acknowledge his hair loss when it was brought to his attention by friends in high school when they teased him or made jokes about it.

When Ralph first noticed that he was losing his hair he was barely eighteen, and "stunned." "I was shocked that it would start so early. I figured I had 30 or 40 years before my hairline would really start receding. And then all of a sudden BOOM!"

Selena said, "It was alarming. And I definitely kept telling myself over and over again, 'It's only hair, and don't get all upset about it'." Angela notes, "Here is a handful of wet hair that just came out because you shampooed it. It was definitely the emotional and mental health aspect of it. It was scary." Roberta, too, said that "it was scary." "I would look in the mirror and say, 'Oh, my God!! Look at my scalp!' And, you know, how many hairs are in this area? And I've started doing that again. I don't do it very often because, I mean, it's too horrifying!"

Simos agrees with Tanner that denial and disbelief — feelings of shock, alarm, even numbness — serve as a "moratorium in time to protect the individual from a flood of emotions and a new reality," feelings that are believed to be normal and appropriate in the face of loss (and psychic trauma), and are regarded as a healthy response. (An unhealthy response, such as prolonged denial and entertaining false hopes, will impede the process of mourning and the final stage of restitution.)[14]

Bargaining

Several of the people that I spoke with referred to bargaining (with a perceived higher power). Walt, who kept a diary through audio taping, said, "Somewhere on my tape I was talking about the experience of losing my hair, and it was like grieving. I went through denial, then bargaining, and somewhere on my tape I was praying. I said, 'Lord, just give me my hair back long enough to find somebody who loves me'."

Yolanda said, "I'd bargain. Say, 'Lord, please give me my hair back. I swear, I'll go to church every Sunday. I'll pay my tithes. Just let me have my hair.' I was bargaining. Believe me, I have done the bargaining. I've done everything. So it's a major loss."

According to Simos, bargaining is a "form of magical thinking wherein a person hopes to influence a higher power through making a promise of certain behavior or sacrifice if he gets his wish." This generally takes place in the early stages of recognizing a loss, and involves an effort to prevent or postpone the inevitable.[15] It seems, too, that bargaining might be an effort to gain control — and having control can reduce stress.[16]

Feelings of Helplessness.

Others spoke of feeling helpless, an overwhelming and debilitating emotion frequently reported in grief. One of the things that made losing his hair so difficult for Walt was the fact that he couldn't do anything about it: "It's like this horrible thing is happening to you. You can't do anything about it and you're going to spend the rest of your life living alone." Bruce said, "I feel kind of powerless. There's nothing you can do there. It kind of gets you down."

Selena said that the worst problem for her was the "control thing." She said:

If you cut your hair short, it's your choice. You did it. But nobody would choose to have those bald spots. There's almost nothing right now that I can do with my hair except comb it straight down. It is something that is happening that you can't do anything about. It's very disturbing.

"There are two aspects to this pain," writes Simos, "the helplessness in longing for that which is irretrievable, and the helplessness in facing the future without that which has been lost."[17] Both aspects seem appropriate for individuals experiencing hair loss: they long to have their hair back, and fear facing the future without it. Yolanda said, "This [my hair] belongs to me. And it's part of me. It's part of my body. And when you start losing it and you didn't ask to lose it or want to lose it there's some control taken away from you and your body." Later during our meeting, she added,

> Part of me that I am supposed to have — unless I choose to cut it off — was gone. Leaving! I had no control over it. Nobody wants to lose anything. I mean, if you're not willing, not ready, to give something up. I mean, we want to be in control of who we are, of our bodies. There is so much out there in the world we have absolutely no control over. Can we please just be in control of our bodies?

"For me," said Mark, "it's definitely a control thing." He said, "Why me? It's like I've got some kind of disease or something. It's like, how could I have no choice in this?" Hattie asked herself a similar question: "Why does it have to happen to me?" She said that she felt angry and more depressed when co-workers asked questions about it, because there was nothing that she could do to stop the hair loss. She felt helpless about the fact that she was losing her hair, not knowing how she was going to hide the baldness, and having people boldly ask her about it.

It's frightening to feel a loss of control over one's body, especially the loss of control over a vital part of one's physical appearance. Why is this so? "A major loss," writes Simos, "is unconsciously a basic threat to survival." Because of the intense relationship between loss and survival, any major loss — or the threat of a loss — sets off in most people a sense of helplessness. Also, the greater the investment of time and emotion in something (such as one's appearance), the greater the reaction is to the loss.[18] Yolanda expressed both anger and helplessness: "I hate it. I really despise it with a passion, and there's not much that I can do. I was losing a part of me that I didn't want to lose. I was grieving."

In the beginning, individuals are usually preoccupied with ideas of how he or she could have prevented the loss, along with feelings of helplessness. The stage of anger in grieving, writes Tanner, generally appears "near the middle or toward the end of the grief cycle."[19]

Anger

When describing his feelings about experiencing hair loss at such a young age, Mark said:

> In high school I know it was a straight up reaction. It was just anger. I've been real defensive about it. It's always been anger. Like in our yearbook, we did these things like bequeaths, you know. And I was bequeathed a membership to the Hair Club for Men. So it was one of the people who did it . . . I didn't think really knew me. So I was mad at them for that.

Grace said, "There would be times when I would just hate my hair as it was growing out and I was like, 'I can't deal with this'." Walt said that "there was a lot of bitterness there." Sheila added:

> I find myself getting defensive when people will ask little questions "too close." But it just happens! And they'll start asking questions, and I just feel it. It's like, "Why? It's none of your business." You know. And I know I shouldn't be like that, but I just get defensive. Real defensive.

Sometimes it's difficult to distinguish between anger and guilt. "What feels like guilt may well be anger which needs to be expressed and dissolved," wrote Jack Miller. Then again, when some individuals are feeling angry, they are only feeling guilty that they didn't do something to prevent the loss.[20]

Guilt and Shame

Several of the people that I spoke with expressed feelings of guilt and shame about their hair loss; others simply blamed themselves for what had happened. Selena said that she felt responsible for her hair loss because she had chosen the type of birth control that she was using. Hattie said, "I know we're not supposed to ask ourselves 'Why? Why did it happen to me?' or, 'What did I do wrong to make this happen?' " Angela appeared to be blaming herself or holding herself accountable for her hair loss when she said, "I think that if I had had the total hair loss, then they [other people] could have said, 'Well, she has cancer. She's in chemo. We won't hold that against her.' "

According to Miller, "Guilt usually runs rampant through all the stages of grief"[21] — a questioning of one's actions, what he or she may have done to cause the loss. Some of the individuals I spoke with actually wondered if they were being punished, thinking that their hair loss was caused by some wrong deed they had committed. Yet others looked for someone else to blame. Yolanda said:

> I think there's a feeling of victimization. The only difference is, though, usually when you feel victimized you can find the perpetrator, and at least deal with it on some level. With alopecia, who do you get to blame? You've got to blame somebody! So you don't get that relief of being able to blame anybody. There's not really anyplace to put hair loss. You own it! It's yours!

Selena said:

> Even now, it's like I'm almost ashamed to go to a beautician because I don't want them to see my bald spots. I keep putting it off and putting it off. And I still have not gone to anybody to do my hair, because of all the shame. You know, it's being women. Even though men feel shame, it's an accepted thing that they will lose their hair at a certain point. People know that male pattern baldness is common. But, even though women do lose their hair, it's something we just don't associate with women. But I do feel ashamed.

Therein lies the agony of shame. Simos defined shame as that feeling which "makes one feel completely exposed, looked at, and sets off the wish to hide, to avoid being seen."[22] (The wish to hide, to keep hair loss a private and personal matter, seems to be a major reaction to hair loss.) Shame is also a typical reaction when one feels that he or she has lost the respect and approval of others.[23] Shame was expressed by the people I spoke with in a variety of ways: some said they felt "shame," several of the women said they felt they were "not living up to society's expectations," others felt they were "looked down upon."

Bruce said that he was trying to hide his baldness because he was "ashamed of it almost" (perhaps related to a perceived loss of manhood or premature aging). Yolanda said that she had felt shame, and she related this to feeling like "less than a woman" and feeling "incomplete." Grace reported "a feeling of being exposed . . . when you lose your hair." Hattie (who has alopecia) said she tried to modify a different hairdo so that her baldness wouldn't be noticeable to people. She added: "I have this problem, and everybody's gonna be looking down on me."

The feelings of being exposed may be related to the fact that it's hard to hide hair loss. Even when one wears a wig, it doesn't take away feelings of shame and insecurity. Kathryn, a young woman who lost her hair as a result of chemotherapy, wrote about her experience:

> You don't have any hair, eyebrows, or eyelashes. I had a very nice wig, so that people would never know that I had lost my hair. But still, I always felt very exposed, very vulnerable. I hated going places where I didn't know anybody. I always felt that people were looking at me, wondering. I hated those kinds of confrontations.[24]

Yolanda's hair was growing back in when I spoke with her. She said that approximately six weeks before our meeting she stopped wearing her wig. When remembering what it felt like to have lost so much hair she said, "I was scared because it really looked bad!" She had to be careful because the remaining bald areas were hard to cover.

> There's nothing to me attractive about losing your hair. So, I felt unattractive. When I got to the point where I had to wear a wig, I worried about my hair [the wig] being pulled off. I used to pull it so tight it gave you a headache. I was afraid it would come off, and I was going to be just standing there.

The feelings of guilt and shame that surround baldness may be linked to its history of being viewed as a negative attribute, even a punishment. For centuries various societies have shaved the heads of traitors, prisoners, and other such offenders.[25] In some countries the hair of an adultress would be cut or shaved, as was the punishment imposed on many French women after World War II who were "suspected of fraternizing with the German occupying troops."[26]

Sadness and Depression

Extreme sadness and depression are generally a reaction to feeling helpless in the face of a painful event. It's the stage of grieving that feels less like a feeling and more like a painful illness.[27] One of the symptoms described by the women I spoke with was crying. "I've cried. I've cried," said Yolanda. "I've cried a lot about losing my hair. I could start crying now if I start thinking about it." Melissa cried several times during our meeting. She said that she asks herself, "Why me?" And added that she has felt "anger" and "sadness" and that she has "been depressed over it." Roberta said, "I was very upset. It was very upsetting."

Grace said,

I was bringing home video tapes on how to tie scarves, and I was practicing, and I was, you know, looking at my hair, and I would be upset. And I would find handfuls, you know. I don't remember a specific time that I cried, but I feel like I must have.

Others simply used words to describe their sadness and depression (particularly the men). When Brad first noticed his receding hairline, ". . . it was depressing, especially at that young of an age. I had kind of expected it. I have a younger brother who was going through the same thing. My father was going through the same thing. So it was no big surprise. But it was very depressing at the time. And as it progressed, it [the depression] got worse." Joy said, "It was devastating." Walt said, "It was really disturbing by the time that I got into college. It was extremely depressing. It was very traumatic for me."

Keeping the Secret

In listening to people talk about their hair loss, the major difference that I found between men and women was the degree of emotional distress. Women voiced stronger feelings and greater sorrow than men. Almost everyone, however, reported efforts to keep their hair loss a secret. Hattie found a beautician who could do a weave-in (a piece of matching false hair is attached with nylon thread to one's own hair.)[28] She said that she would get up in the morning and say to herself, 'What in the world am I gonna do with my hair for the day? So I began to get more and more depressed, you know, trying to hide it with bobby pins, pulling hair over and stuff. That was when I had to get a weave-in done."

"Wigs were my solution," said Yolanda. "And there's nothing like walking around with a wig and praying that nobody pulls it off, or it doesn't fall off. There's not a perfect-fitting wig, like everybody says. I wore a wig for two years, and I hated it. I really did."

Angela said that she bought a wig from the Cancer Society, but she didn't feel comfortable wearing it. "I eventually went to a drugstore, and they had these 'kerchief things' and I got several of those." Later in the interview, she added, "Even now, I still have a very strong desire to cover my head, even though to a normal person, you don't realize that I have lost hair. Only I know this. I knew what I had before, and I know how much is gone."

Prior to her surgery, chemotherapy, and subsequent hair loss, Renata Polt had been a daily swimmer. It was difficult facing her friends in the locker room with a bald head, but she wasn't going to give it up. On her first day back she entered the locker room with a scarf covering her bare head and immediately went into a toilet stall. Feeling the privacy of this small, closed-in space, she uncovered her head, donned her bathing suit, and struggled with the bathing cap. After her swim she covered her head with a towel, carefully removed the cap, then wrapped the towel around her head.Once again she sought the privacy of the toilet stall to dry off, get dressed, and don her scarf.[29]

The loss of one's hair — such a vital part of a woman's appearance — is troubling. The implications of this loss, what it means in terms of having a full and enjoyable life, are enormous. Women will carefully guard their secret, decide who they can risk sharing their secret with, and determine how close those relationships will be. Selena said the only person who knew that she was losing her hair was her husband. She said that she never lost the hair on top of her head, and she was able to comb it forward and wear a headband or a hat. She said, "my friends don't know; just my husband knows, just my husband. Because I really didn't want anybody else to see." She said that it takes a lot of time to arrange her hair to cover the balding areas, and this has had a major effect on her life. "It wasn't always 'time' either. No. I keep saying 'time,' and it wasn't always 'time.' Sometimes, I guess, it was kind of disheartening. And, you know, it's still disheartening."

Grace used scarves as an alternative headcovering.

> I remember feeling really self-conscious about doing that. It bothered me . . . because I didn't ever like the way it looked. I felt like I looked really, really sick . . . sicker at that point than I ever had when I was really sick. And here I was coming back to work . . . and, you know . . . having to see everybody again.

Mark wore a baseball cap to the interview, as did Ralph. Both men kept their caps on during the meetings, and both indicated that they kept their heads covered most of the time. Ralph shared that his hair loss may have hurt his career on occasions because he felt so self-conscious about it. Bruce said that at first he wore baseball caps, and then he tried various haircuts. He described everyone's feelings accurately when he said: "You don't want people to see that you have hair loss. You don't want other people to see it!"

The feelings expressed here are all part of grieving the loss of an important body part, and equally important, a loss of freedom: the freedom to be comfortable in the world and to know that there is nothing — at least, nothing visible — to hide. For women experiencing hair loss, it's a life of fear, the fear of being found out. The feelings that men experience are also about fear, the fear of being rejected, especially by the opposite sex.

Acceptance

"The grief process has a rhythm all its own, " writes Miller. "Like the seasons of the year, there is a winter of our personal lives, a time when we feel fallow and cold within, and a springtime of deep joy."[30] Several of the people I spoke with felt that they were approaching a new season. They seemed to be resolving their grief, and finally accepting their hair loss. Walt said, "Going bald has really forced me to look at who I am, and to either accept myself or reject myself, and I've accepted myself. When Cathy [his wife] came into my life it was plainly evident to me that that was all taken care of. And so that relieved a lot of the fear in me, and it allowed me to believe that my hair wasn't all that meaningful."

Renata Polt spoke to her oncologist about the slow regrowth of her hair. "Let's wait and see," he said. "And if it doesn't come in, well, I'll refer you to the best wig maker in town." Now in the process of resolving her hair loss, Renata replied, "Never!"

> By now I was wearing berets only when it was cold outside, always removing them indoors. I was so happy to be alive, to have my body and to have it more or less intact, that I valued every part of it in ways I'd never dreamed of, even when I was younger and better-looking. My head was going to be part of me. Hair, or no hair.[31]

"I've been like, I'm losing my hair, that's right, I'm cool," said Bret. "I'll get respect now, by God." Humor seemed to be helping him a lot with the process of accepting his hair loss. He added, "I deal with it better than I used to."

Dave was less emotional about his hair loss than many of the others that I spoke with. Toward the end of the interview he added, "Hair seems to me to be little more than physical attractiveness." He indicated a level of acceptance of his baldness when he said, "Other than making me look younger and somewhat more attractive, I don't see what difference it would make. That is the only thing that has bothered me, and it has bothered me a lot less as time has gone on."

Ralph, too, alluded to accepting his hair loss when he said,

> It's funny. Growing up, my father did not take a lot of inter-

est in a lot of things that I did, unless I was in trouble. And, you know, the kind of family life I had was very difficult to get any attention whatsoever. So I just marched along as best I could. And I guess the point I'm trying to make is that if I lose my hair, I lose my hair. You know, I'm going to be me, no matter what.

Several of the people that I spoke with, however, may have more difficulty resolving their loss. "It will get progressively worse," said Bruce, "so that's depressing. It's an ongoing thing. It's a long, long cycle that is really never over." Melissa said, "I don't see how I can be used to it. I deal with it. I go on, do what I need to do. I try not to dwell on it. I go through spells sometimes when it really, really gets to me."

Yolanda said, "It's just an overwhelming feeling of just being vulnerable; just feeling scared and nervous. You're tense, you're unhappy, you're not comfortable. You don't feel whole. You don't feel complete. I felt some despair."

Mark said, "I really think the thing is, it's [hair loss] a part of me and I don't want it to be. And I think that's where it comes down. And I'd rather be remembered for something else." He said, "It's almost like, you know, I'm vulnerable. Because at any time somebody could bring up some kind of hair comment. And I don't like that. I don't like being vulnerable to something like that."

Sheila said that her mother saved her hair because she thought that it might help in trying to figure out if her hair loss was genetic, or the doctors might need it at some point to identify a cause (and cure). Sheila said that she herself wants to know — if she has children — "what are the chances that they would have this problem. Because, unless I knew I would have boys . . . boys probably could handle it a lot better than a girl. And I know what I go through. It is hard enough for me. And to think that I would have a girl and she would have to go through what I go through."

Roxane Silver and Camille Wortman said that for many individuals a traumatic experience involving loss is never really resolved, just tolerated in a more peaceful manner. They say that some people simply learn to live with their loss. Realistically, we can't expect a truly painful experience to be erased from the memory, especially one that is life altering. To reflect on an agonizing event from time to time — and voice sad feelings about it — is not a sign of weakness or instability. It can simply be the way the trauma is dealt with.[32]

The inner life changes that result from losing one's hair are profound: coping with feeling different than others, unattractive, undesirable — feelings that are generally dealt with in private. On an intensely personal level, hair loss seems to disconnect people from society and from humanity in general. (Keeping one's hair loss a secret — keeping any secret — automatically creates a separation from others.) As Brad said, "It's not just hair. It is so emotional." It's the fear of being discarded, of not belonging; the loss of a youthful, sensual appearance; the loss of body image; it's the loss of feeling secure and confident when around the opposite sex.

HAIR LOSS AND THE LOSS OF SEXUAL ATTRACTIVENESS

Most of the people that I spoke with felt self-conscious about their hair loss — around friends, family members, co-workers, even strangers. As mentioned, almost everyone made attempts to hide their baldness. Women, especially, lived in fear that their secret would be discovered. The strongest feelings surrounding hair loss, however, appear to be connected to the role that hair plays in the rituals of dating, courtship, and, in some cases, marriage.

Melissa revealed how she isolates herself from men and distances herself from the world. She longs for her hair to grow back, and she wants a normal life. Hattie didn't want her husband to know. Walt's feelings about his hair loss appeared to be based on a fear of being rejected by women: "I think the whole thing for me was tied up in a loss of self-worth and the likelihood of spending my life alone." He said, "I think that the only way that I really ever overcame that was in finding a woman who would love me for who I was."

> I always tell women, "It's like, if you had this disease that
> makes you put on one ounce of weight everyday and nobody
> notices it from day to day . . . but over the next five years
> you're going to put on 60 pounds, and you're never going to
> be able to shake it, and it's always going to be there, and you
> can't do anything about it."

Walt said that his previous girlfriend was upset about his hair loss:

> I would bring it up. I'd say, "Are you still going to like me
> when I'm bald?" And she'd go, "Yeah, but I still wish you
> had hair." You know, that was a weird situation to be in, and
> I'm glad I'm not in it anymore. It was really depressing. Be-
> cause what I wanted her to say desperately was, "I don't
> care. I'm gonna love you anyway." And she didn't. And that
> was exactly what I did not need to hear at that time.

Clearly, the biggest concern for Walt about losing his hair was
about being unattractive and not being successful at finding a suitable mate.

> If you've already found someone who loves you uncondi-
> tionally, then that's okay ... but the idea for me of going bald
> before I found that was really scary. The thing for me was
> that I felt like if I was bald, then I wouldn't be attractive.
> And if I wasn't attractive, I'd never find anybody who would
> love me. And if I didn't have anybody love me, I'd spend the
> rest of my life lonely.

Don said, "One of the major factors for me is, do I think this
[hair loss] is going to preclude me from something that I really would
like, which would be to be in a relationship that's gonna last."

Throughout the interview with Bret, he stressed that his hair loss
had been a bigger problem for him (emotionally) during the years
that he was a single man and dating. He said, "It does effect you if
you're single a lot more than if you're married. I mean, it did me.
Because it does affect your self-confidence a little bit as far as dealing with women or just dealing with people in general." He said that
he does consider himself less physically attractive because of his
hair loss.

Clearly, hair is a sexual object — perhaps one reason why we
are obsessed with it. It is equated with physical attractiveness, sensuality, romance, virility, femininity and masculinity. Within certain
religious groups it is removed to minimize sexual attractiveness. If
anyone doubts the value that is placed on hair in our society, "simply
leafing through newspaper or magazine articles and advertisements

will show just how important hair is to the general population," say Sadick and Richardson.[33] Consequently, the loss of hair will cast fear and doubt on a person's self-esteem and sexual-esteem: a fear of rejection, of being alone, of not being desirable or lovable. (One's physical appearance generally plays a role in these fearful feelings, as physical attractiveness is often reported as the most important factor in dating or in finding a partner.)[34] When an individual loses his or her hair, all of these fears are provoked and the losses are extensive. To make matters worse, it is a frightening, lonely, and silent mourning.

FINDING SUPPORT

Many of the people that I spoke with did not look for help or support with their grieving, saying that they feared their feelings would be judged as superficial, vain, and self-centered. Consequently, they kept their pain to themselves. This isn't unusual. Silver and Wortman said that the "view that one's behavior is inappropriate may prevent persons from seeking support from others in their time of distress."[35] The truth is that many people with hair loss are given the message that their feelings are silly and unreasonable. Melissa said that some of her family members said that she "should be used to it by now." They assume that her hair loss doesn't bother her anymore since she doesn't talk about it. She expressed ongoing emotional pain when she tearfully said that "it's not something that you get used to."

There are several ways that a person experiencing pain over hair loss can get help. The first is to find a compassionate therapist. The second is to join a support group. The third is to search the Internet. Finding a psychotherapist isn't difficult; finding the right psychotherapist can be. It's important for anyone considering psychotherapy to interview several therapists and to look for the following behavioral traits: empathy, therapeutic support, good listening skills, a good sense of humor. Above all it is important to find a therapist who validates his or her client's emotional experience. As Silver and Wortman point out, "It behooves the health-care professional to legitimize the feelings and reactions that commonly occur among people who have encountered negative life events."[36] A support group can also help with this aspect of therapy, as no one will understand feelings as well as those who are having the same experience. Support groups are generally advertised, and almost all psychotherapists are aware of the different groups held in the community. One can even find comfort, and oftentimes a group, on the Internet. This method of finding support is perhaps the least threatening, and can be a good beginning toward discovering that one's feelings are indeed normal.

Loss is an essential part of our existence, say the experts. It seems to be what life is all about. Fighting it only prolongs the process. Ever so slowly, we have to say good-bye to many aspects of our lives: the grand ideas of how we think we should look, how life should be, our fantasies of everlasting love, of producing perfect children, our youth. These events occur naturally. They are inevitable losses. Losing one's hair, however, is an untimely event. It is an agonizing and wretched experience and involves many more feelings than concern about body image, as there are many other losses that come about as a result of this drastic change in one's appearance. Each loss must be acknowledged and dealth with. As Simos said — and as the people that I spoke with indicated — loss of a part of the body can be as devastating as the loss of a loved one.

Regardless, we do not rise out of grief the same person we were before. Grief requires something of us: to endure our mourning, to develop confidence in getting through the difficult times, to mature, and to develop a stronger character. It asks that we face our loss as a challenge in life, rather than a problem. It asks that we trust: trust life, trust ourselves, and trust others.[37] It tells us that life is about being humbled, not humiliated. We assign a value to each part of our body. We value some parts more than others[38] — the vital organs, the sexual organs, and especially the parts of our body that we show to the world. Our hair is one of those parts.

CHAPTER SEVEN

SURVIVAL SKILLS

Nine Techniques for Coping with Hair Loss

"Life is hard," I reflected while lunching with Ann and Meggan, my good friends and colleagues.

"We know this better than most," Meggan replied. "Our work demands that we sit with painful and intense emotions, mostly sorrow."

> *The outer forms of our lives can change in an instant, but the inner reorientation that brings us back into a vital relation to people and activity takes time.*
> — William Bridges

The dialogue flowed — a typical conversation among three compassionate psychotherapists sharing a meal in a quiet, dimly lit restaurant.

"The best way to help our clients face the ambiguities and uncertainties of life, the distressing, unexpected events," Meggan added, "is to offer healthy ways to cope; to teach them skills that help them through the difficult times that inevitably appear in everyone's lifetime."

We solemnly and supportively agreed.

When clients are faced with troublesome situations — situations over which they have no control — the therapist's aim is to help them survive their trauma without making matters worse; to assist them in how to remain physically, spiritually, psychologically, and emotionally intact until they can make it on their own. Losing one's hair can be such an event. For many it is a traumatic, lonely, and emotionally devastating experience.

Hence, what follows is a set of proven skills borrowed from all walks of life — spiritual, psychological, philosophical — each intended to help one survive the emotional experience of hair loss. Each skill is presented with a *premise* (rationale behind its use), an *example* (how others have used it), and an *anticipated outcome* (what can be expected as a result of its use).

ATTITUDE IS EVERYTHING

Albert Ellis, the founder of Rational Emotive Therapy, says that it isn't what happens to us in life that causes our distress, it's how we view it. In other words, no experience has an assessed value *in and of itself*. We, individually, assign value to everything.[1]

Our value systems (from which we form opinions and decisions) are not necessarily our own, however. Much of what we view as fair or unfair, right or wrong, good or bad, we have adopted from our families, friends, teachers, advisors, mentors, and from society as a whole. Hence, each of us runs the risk of falling prey to *group thought*. "Obviously, then," writes Ellis, "we have *some* degree of choice and control over our responses to various situations."[2] These responses or reactions to life events are what we shall call *attitude*.

According to Robert Baron and Donn Byrne, authors of *Social Psychology: Understanding Human Interaction*, reactions (or attitudes) can take many forms, but most fall under three major headings: *affective, cognitive,* and *behavioral*. This means that an individual losing his or her hair will often react with feelings (*affective*), thoughts (*cognitive*), and action (*behavior*). Most would agree that our feelings and thoughts generally affect how we handle situations.[3] This is especially true with cognition (one's thinking). Because thoughts guide perceived reality,[4] it is important to recognize the power of thoughts when one is worrying about hair loss. One's perspective, or thinking — like telling oneself that people will reject you — can lead to certain behaviors (i.e., isolation). Whatever your thoughts are about hair loss, they will ultimately determine your feelings about it — and, subsequently, how you react.

Research shows that the opposite can also be true: An individual's behavior can, over time, change his or her feelings and thoughts.[5] A skill (*changing your current emotion by acting opposite to that emotion*) taught in dialectical behavioral therapy (DBT) explains this theory well. According to Marsha Linehan, the founder of DBT, when you act opposite to what you're feeling, "your behavior or actions communicate to your brain, and the effect is a slow but steady change in your emotions."[6] When using this particular skill it's important to keep three things in mind: (1) it will work if your reaction to the situation is not realistic; (2) suppressing, masking, or hiding your emotions is not the goal — only to act contrary to what you're feeling; and (3) you must truly want to change the emotion.[7]

Premise: A negative attitude about losing one's hair can be altered somewhat by changing one's actions (behaving as if one truly isn't bothered by it).

Example: Jojuan Lamorreaia, who lost her hair to alopecia areata, said that it took her about thirty tries before she walked out of her house without her wig on. For ten years she had been a slave to synthetic materials. Finally, she refused to "hide in shame and embarrassment" over a situation in which she had no control. On that particular day she realized that she was much too bothered about public opinion. She didn't wear her wig. Yes, people gawked and cars slowed down, but some yelled, "Go on, sister!" Now, Jojuan never wears a wig, and she likes her different, unique look.[8]

Expected Outcome: By committing oneself to a desired behavior (an exposure-based procedure), one's unrealistic feelings about a situation will dissipate.

This writer is in no way suggesting that individuals who are balding should appear in public bareheaded. The recommendation is simply to assess your attitude about losing your hair; if it is sufficiently negative that it causes you distress, or limits your life in any way, it's time for an attitude adjustment.

1. Determine your desired goal (how would you like to feel about

your hair loss?);

2. Identify the behavior that would demonstrate the desired attitude; and

3. Act accordingly.

Changing one's attitude about hair loss isn't exactly simple. However, success is just around the corner if one can do three things: view it as a challenge rather than a problem, remain committed to one's activities in life, and take control — all these steps work against feelings of powerlessness.[9] Willie Jolley, a motivational speaker, supports these approaches. For every problem in life, he says, "There can be a defining moment that begins the transformation process and turns the tide from a negative direction to a positive direction."[10] The transformation begins with a decision — the decision to view one's hair loss as an opportunity (not a problem); to remain committed to living one's life (not alienated); and to take charge (rather than feel helpless).[11]

Humor

"I've cried a lot about losing my hair," said Yolanda. "And I joke about it a lot — mainly because it kind of deflects the painful feelings." Yolanda is correct in her thinking. Exercising positive emotions (i.e., laughing) sets off a process in the body that wards off negativity. Humor, for example, reduces tension, increases energy, and provides a sense of well-being.[12] "Laughter mobilizes our best feelings," writes a cancer/hair loss survivor. It "helps you breathe deep, relaxes your body and mind, and sets your spirit free."[13]

By suggesting humor as a skill to cope, I am not asking anyone to trivialize the experience of hair loss. The rationale behind using comic relief is that it humanizes the situation. It creates a "less intimidating and scary" environment writes Selma Schimmel. Laughing "allows people to come closer to you."[14] It helps us engage with life and helps us feel less isolated.

Men especially find humor in hair loss. In his book, *Bald Men Always Come Out on Top*, Dave Beswick sites "101 Ways to Use Your Head and Win with Skin." Beswick debunks myths about hair loss. He points out the positive aspects of not having any hair; he identifies famous sports figures, actors, writers, musicians, religious figures, and world leaders who are (or were) bald. His book provides all-around good humor for those who are losing their hair.[15]

The skill of accessing humor may be hard to accomplish during the early stages of hair loss. It's hard to laugh — though not impossible — when one is grieving a loss. And forcing it can only make matters worse. However, when the time is right, remember:

Premise: Laughter is psychologically healing. It can lend comfort and reassurance in difficult situations.[16] Simply put, humor can lighten a painful experience.

Example: A young, attractive cancer/hair loss survivor said that she felt "very self-conscious about being bald" when she was going through chemotherapy. She didn't want to wear a wig, so she chose hats. She was getting a lot of attention from cute guys when she was out for her walks. "You know, guys would drive by and honk. One time this guy shouted an obscenity, so I tipped my hat to him. You should have seen his face. That was hysterical."[17]

Expected Outcome: Humor makes life less problematic. It's brings relief; helps one take a break. "It removes the dark lens that you see your life through and gives you a lighter lens that gives you clarity," says Loretta LaRoche. Essentially, humor helps you create the next higher version of yourself.[18]

Conquer Your Fear

Fear can be helpful (i.e., a warning of impending danger), or it can be a completely useless feeling. Joseph Wolpe, author of *Our Useless Fears*, says that "useful fears function largely as a signaling device." Fear is worthless, he says, "when, instead of being helpful, it gets in the way."[19] The most common fears experienced by individuals with hair loss are the fear of being stared at (the focus of everyone's attention), the fear of being different, and the fear of being rejected.[20]

Although fear surrounding hair loss seems useless, disruptive, and limiting, the individuals that I spoke with believed that their feelings were appropriate and reasonable. Most blamed it on society — especially the media — indicating that being bald is not generally considered attractive by the masses. Bret said, "Everyone you see on TV that's supposed to be desirable or whatever has a full head of hair." "It's purely social," said Jake. "Sexually aggressive or sexually open women tend to like men with really long hair." (He associated this tendency with the popularity and success of certain, long-haired, male rock stars.) Don also blamed his fear on social norms, saying, "There's an attitude in society that being bald is not attractive." And along with acknowledging the media's role in portraying hair as a required, sensual asset, Sheila, Roberta, and Yolanda recalled that a great deal of time and energy was spent on their hair when they were children, instilling in them the belief that a woman's hair is especially important. "It's societal" and "it's cultural," said Roberta. "All those commercials on television."[21]

So, how does one overcome a fear that seems both rational and irrational? First, by identifying the basis (or origin) of the fear regarding hair loss.[22] Second, by examining the reality of danger involved (this is usually what fear is about).[23] Third, by putting into practice several skills designed to help individuals overcome fear and anxiety: engage in positive denial, do a systematic desensitization, practice mindful breathing, develop a daily exercise routine, and, if all else fails, feel the fear and do it anyway.

Positive Denial

Sigmund Freud was one of the earlier theorists who identified denial as a means of coping. He proposed that fear (or anxiety) could be relieved temporarily by simply ignoring the cause of the fear.[24] In more recent times another noted theorist, Dr. Richard Lazarus, proposed that in certain situations — especially harmless situations — intentionally choosing *denial* may be the healthiest strategy for coping. "My own research on how people actually deal with life crises," says Lazarus, "has brought me around to the view that illusion and self-deception can have positive value in a person's psychological economy."[25] Because hair loss is a physically harmless experience, positive denial can be practiced in any number of ways, depending on the basis of the fear. For example, if the fear is about being the focus of attention (i.e., stared at) while in public, one can simply concentrate on the task at hand and consciously deny that anyone may be looking.

Lazarus suggests that realistic (and encouraging) self statements can help when first practicing the skill of positive denial.[26] An example would be saying to oneself, "It's probably normal that I am a little afraid of going out in public the first time after losing my hair, even if I do have a wig on. I'll get used to it. No one will notice that this isn't my real hair."

Systematic Desensitization

Systematic desensitization, or graduated calming, is a process by which one can become less vulnerable (or sensitive) to whatever is triggering the fear (i.e., fear of one's wig or hair piece falling off in public). The process is outlined systematically, and only after the fear is conquered at a lower level can he or she move on to the next, slightly more difficult level. It's important to note that before tackling each step, one should be in a relaxed and confident state of mind. (You may wish to see a psychotherapist to guide you through exposure therapy.)[27]

Mindful Breathing

Breathing fast — even holding or suppressing one's breath — is a common response to fear or any uncomfortable feeling. Our emotions are so closely linked to our breath, says Andy Caponigro, "that we can actually change how we feel simply by changing how we breathe."[28] When using this skill, attention is brought totally (and completely) to one's breathing, with each breath being observed and described in any number of ways: One can breathe slowly while counting each breath (i.e., one, two, three); or say, "I am breathing in, I am breathing out."[29] Some individuals use the 7-11 method of mindful breathing: Slowly counting to seven while breathing in, and mindfully counting to eleven while breathing out.

Mindful breathing is a form of meditation in that it gives you something to focus on. The trick is to stay focused. Herbert Benson suggests that when you do get distracted — and you will — simply return to the way you were observing your breath.[30]

All mindfulness skills (focusing on the moment) are effective. I am choosing mindful breathing simply because breathing is a constant; it is always with us, and it is easily focused on.

Daily Physical Exercise

Daily physical exercise "can improve your stamina and boost your spirits," writes Stacy Taylor.[31] It can help one feel emotionally centered, more relaxed, and simply better equipped to face the challenges that await an individual experiencing hair loss.

Anyone committed to a regular exercise routine can verify the positive effects of a good workout. Tension, anxiety, even anger seem to drift away after a power walk, jogging, running, or lifting weights. "The effect of exercise is immediate," writes Dr. Michael Norden. "Research indicates that twenty to forty minutes of aerobic exercise temporarily lessens anxiety and improves mood, an effect that lasts several hours."[32]

The body is always in motion, even when asleep: The heart beats, the diaphragm forces air in and out of the lungs, the body sometimes tosses and turns, seeking a more comfortable position. The commitment to exercise on a regular basis simply helps the body fulfill its function more effectively.[33] It can also build self-confidence, an important ingredient in conquering one's fears.

Feel the Fear and Do It Anyway

This method of overcoming fear is similar to the opposite to emotion action skill discussed earlier; the difference rests in how one approaches the uncomfortable feeling of fear or anxiety. Fear itself isn't the problem, says Susan Jeffers, it's "how we hold the fear." One can hold fear "from a position of power (i.e., choice, energy and action)," or "from a position of pain (i.e., helplessness, depression and paralysis)." The trick in managing fear is to move oneself "from a position of pain to a position of power." (Fear is inconsequential if one is experiencing it from a position of power.)[34] The central feeling when one is in a position of pain is helplessness. Taking control of the situation, then, is essential.

Jeffers says that fear in most cases is an educational problem. Fear — the kind that gets in one's way — can be "unlearned," she says, with courage and commitment, and by shifting one's thinking. The tools she offers are based on the simple truth that fear is a part of life, "rather than a barrier to success."[35] Hence, as long as one is taking risks, pushing forward toward goals, striving to grow and improve one's life, fear will be a constant companion.[36] Accepting this idea about fear is the first step toward overcoming it.

Premise: Fear arises according to one's appraisal of an event, how easily one can adapt to what's happening, and how one is holding the fear. If one's fear is unrealistic or unreasonable — even if one has no control over a threatening event — using certain coping skills can minimize the sometimes paralyzing feeling of fear.

Example: Sheila, who as a child was diagnosed with alopecia universalis, said that things "eased up a bit" (found her personal power?) when she went to college. She said to herself, "Hey, this is something I can't help. I didn't cause this. And if people don't understand that's their problem. I'm able to deal with it, and I know I'm fine!"[37]

Expected Outcome: Without irrational fears about hair loss, you can exercise more freedom, worry less, and find greater enjoyment in life.

Do Something Pleasurable Every Day

Sadly, in this day and time, *doing something pleasurable on a daily basis* is a skill that needs to be taught to many individuals — mostly adults. Enjoying life a little each day (or *creative selfishness*,[38] as Louden sees it) should continue from childhood, through adolescence, the teen years, and right into adulthood. Realistically, however, daily pleasures (for many) are buried beneath work, family, and the many responsibilities that most adults face everyday. To lead a healthy, well-rounded life, pleasurable leisure activities on a regular basis are necessary. An added benefit is that negative emotions (i.e., fear, worry) decrease in relation to the number of positive experiences one enjoys.[39]

This means that negative feelings about hair loss can be minimized in relation to the number of positive experiences you seek out in your life. Please note that recreational activities do not have to be dramatic or costly — they can range from reading a good book to purchasing a new wig to attending the opera.

Premise: One can increase positive feelings by increasing the number of positive experiences in one's life.[40]

Example: My good friend Meggan often reflects on the summer of 1990, and remembers how happy she was. "I was trying to figure it out," she said, "and then I realized I felt happy because I was doing everything that I thoroughly enjoy. I read, wrote music, met friends in town [walking distance from her house] for meals, wrote letters, attended performances [both music and drama.] I indulged myself in simple pleasures."

Expected Outcome: Negative feelings (i.e., fear, mad, sadness) about one's hair loss will decrease according to the number of positive experiences one has.[41]

Tend to Your Basic Needs

Attending to your basic needs is not only important as a health requirement, it is crucial to how well you cope with negative feelings about losing your hair. Eating well-balanced meals, getting enough sleep, developing an exercise routine, finding productive work, enjoying leisure activities, nurturing and appreciating one's relationships — all are important for "brain maintenance," reports Edward M. Hallowell.[42] One can simply cope with life's difficulties more effectively if basic survival needs are met.

Tending to one's health needs as an effective way of coping has long been practiced within support groups of recovering alcoholics (Alcoholics Anonymous, or AA). The word HALT is given as an acronym in order to remember: Never let yourself get too Hungry, too Angry, too Lonely, or too Tired. AA members know that they are much more likely to reach for a drink — and we, as a species, are much more likely to be controlled (or affected) by negative feelings about hair loss — if our basic needs are not met.

Premise: Maintaining good health practices, say Salvatore Maddi and Suzanne Kobasa, is a resistance resource "that has a buffering effect by decreasing strain." Exercise, good nutrition, leisure activities, etc., all aim at improving one's ability to cope with unwanted events.[43]

Example: Helen did her best to take good care of herself. She said: "I'm trying to stay as natural in my body maintenance as possible. I try to not take drugs, I take vitamins, eat very little meat, buy organic vegetables, and that kind of thing. I don't eat a lot of sugar, I don't eat a lot of fat." She said she liked to swim; said she got an adequate amount of rest; spoke of ongoing contact with several devoted friends; indicated that she was enjoying life in spite of her hair loss. She was also embarking on a new career (she was in graduate school).[44]

Expected Outcome: One is more relaxed, and less affected by negative feelings about hair loss if basic needs are met.

Most importantly, good nutrition is vital for individuals experiencing hair loss — especially if the loss is a result of chemotherapy. Poor nutrition due to vomiting or loss of appetite can lead to dull and lifeless hair,[45] and even further loss as a result of protein deficiency. Individuals suffering from anorexia nervosa frequently report hair loss, a result of malnutrition.[46]

TAKE CARE OF BUSINESS

"Take care of business," means that on a daily basis we do the necessary chores that keep life on track — pay bills, grocery shop, plan meals, do laundry — along with any small task that we have been avoiding (i.e., cleaning out a closet). Marsha Linehan calls this "mastery." She says that when individuals engage in activities that "build a sense of self-efficacy and competence," they are less vulnerable to negative emotions.[47] Hacking away at a list of chores also gives people a sense of control over their lives.

The issue of *control* — especially for individuals experiencing hair loss — can be monumental. As Selena remarked, [hair loss] is "a *you're not in control* kind of issue." Most all of the people that I spoke with brought up feelings of *no control*. Walt spoke for everyone when he said, "It's happening, you don't like it, and there's nothing you can do about it."[48]

Being a psychotherapist, I am well aware of the paralyzing effects that can accompany feelings of helplessness. The belief (or realization) that one has no control over a situation — one that matters a great deal — often leads to depression, anxiety, and sometimes despair. It appears to be the reason why many individuals seek therapy. Helping clients feel in control of their lives (in any way) seems to help enormously.

Premise: Accomplishing small, but important tasks in life helps us feel better about ourselves, helps us feel like functional beings, gives us a sense of control.

Example: Bret is married and has two children. He indicated that simply being involved in family activities (i.e., yard work, house maintenance, Little League) has helped him worry less about losing his hair. "Its not such a big deal to me anymore since I'm married, have kids, and trying to keep up with all of those responsibilities. I'm busy!"[49]

Expected Outcome: Involving yourself in daily tasks — no matter how mundane — will bring about a sense of accomplishment, and will help you feel in charge of your life. (Such tasks will also distract you from problems over which you have no control.)

Comfort Yourself

Self-nurturing and/or *comforting the self* are defined by Jennifer Louden as "having the courage to pay attention to your needs," finding comforting ways to "fortify yourself," and above all, to accept yourself. "Self-care begins and ends with ourselves," she writes.[50]

It's completely up to us.

Linehan, too, stresses the importance of soothing the self, especially when one is experiencing intense, unpleasant emotions. She advocates healing attention to one (or all) of the senses: seeing, hearing, smelling, tasting, and touching.[51] This means that should you be experiencing unpleasant emotions in regard to your hair loss, you can recenter yourself by nurturing yourself in one of the following ways: prepare your favorite dish — one that you enjoy smelling and eating; listen to your favorite symphony (or rhythm and blues) album while bathing in a hot tub surrounded by scented candles; apply a favorite lotion to your skin; listen to a relaxation tape while resting.

Premise: Being gentle and kind to ourselves helps us tolerate everyday life, survive unpleasant experiences, and feel attended to.[52] Soothing the self in any way helps one feel less lonely, builds confidence, and gives one a sense of control.

Example: Melissa, who lives alone, looks forward to going home at night. She draws the shades, takes off her wig, and lets her scalp breathe. She puts on loose, comfortable clothing, plays her favorite music, and she enjoys a good meal. Later she soaks in hot bath water that has been scented with a favorite fragrance. Around 10 PM she falls asleep reading a good novel.

Expected Outcome: Taking control of our comfort needs (rather than expecting another to provide these luxurious and refreshing moments) renews the spirit, and helps us feel relaxed and in control.

GET INVOLVED

Getting involved can be achieved in many different ways. Grace stepped back into life by donning a scarf and returning to work in the hospital. Helen had been accepted into a graduate program in the School of Public Health. Regardless of extensive hair loss, almost all of the individuals I spoke with were involved in life in productive ways.

Some individuals experiencing baldness choose to involve them-selves in work (even volunteer work) that surrounds the issue of hair loss itself. Some become active in cancer organizations, assisting cancer survivors who have lost their hair. Others participate in sup-port groups or on-line chat rooms or offer supportive assistance (usu-ally through their physician) to those who are losing their hair.

If a support group is not available in your area, you could start one. Remember that a support group can begin with only two people. One single confidante can bring an end to feelings of isolation, can lend new perspectives, and often give helpful advice. As the group grows in number, so do the rewards. In a caring, supportive environ-ment, we tend to reveal our innermost thoughts and feelings. In an atmosphere of trust we can learn more about ourselves and come to know and appreciate ourselves. George Leonard and Michael Murphy tell us that, "Through the growing self-acceptance that is encour-aged by the presence of empathic listeners, our wounds can be healed and our capacities developed more freely."[53]

Marsha Linehan calls the act of being helpful "contributing" and identifies it as a skill to be used when one is experiencing considerable stress. Her rationale is that by performing kind deeds for another, we are less obsessed with our own pain and sorrow. Contributing can also in-crease "a sense of meaning in life" and enhance our self-respect.[54]

Premise: Involving ourselves with others (in charitable ways) helps us feel better. It also distracts us from our misery.

Example: Angela hopes to become a care-giver so that she can in-volve herself with others (especially women) who are experi-encing hair loss. She plans to enter the nursing profession.

Expected Outcome: "Those who serve others in love and kindness," say Leonard and Murphy, "enjoy better health and live longer."[55]

REMEMBER: YOU ARE NOT YOUR HAIR

"Your body helps define who you are," writes Stacy Taylor. Hence, when one's body changes dramatically — as with hair loss — it's important to remember that your body is only "part of you."[56]

Your hair only *helps* define who you are; you are not your hair. As Bret said: "It's just part of accepting who you are as a person. It's just one component of who you are." In spite of his hair loss, Ralph, too, seemed to have grasped a sense of himself: "If I lose all of my hair I lose my hair. I'm me, and I'm still going to be me no matter what."[57]

Grace, who temporarily lost her hair as the result of a serious illness, was grateful to be alive and functioning. She was able to put her hair loss in perspective and acknowledge that she, herself, was important — that she, as a human being, *mattered*. "Relative to what I'd been through, this was so minor. I was just glad to be alive. I could walk and that was my big thing."[58]

What I am talking about here is reassessing our values; accepting the loss of an important body part; finding a deeper truth; looking below the surface literally and committing to a different reality. The more clearly we see reality, writes M. Scott Peck, "the better equipped we are to deal with the world."[59] In recognizing that we are more than our hair, in acknowledging our inner strengths, we can overcome the emotional experience of hair loss — at least to the degree that we can feel good about ourselves again.

Premise: By working on acceptance (i.e., accepting that your hair is only part of who you are), by appreciating the other parts of your body (especially the vital organs), you can put your hair loss in perspective and lead a satisfying, happy, and productive life.

Example: Taylor recommends an exercise to help make peace with your body (this includes your self image): Find a comfortable place to sit and relax. Take a few breaths, and calm your body. Next, take a couple of minutes to scan your body from head to toe. As you do this, notice all of the parts of your body that are working fine with no help from anyone. Visualize your eyes seeing, your lungs breathing, your heart pumping blood throughout your system. As you do this, express appreciation to your body. Say, for instance, "I appreciate that my kidneys are functioning." Thank the different parts of your body for working so hard to keep you alive. Say to your body, "I know that you struggle sometimes. But you're doing the best you can. Thank you for the effort."[60]

Expected Outcome: Recognizing that you are more than your hair and honoring other parts of your body, will help you appreciate who you really are.

⤳

Each of the nine skills offered presents an opportunity to move beyond the process of balding and improve one's self-esteem. The skills center around improving one's attitude, using humor, overcoming fears, engaging in pleasurable activities on a daily basis, tending to one's basic needs, attending to chores, comforting oneself, and getting involved in helping others.

Recognizing that *attitude is everything* is paramount in accomplishing the task of putting one's hair loss in perspective. Using humor simply lessens the emotional intensity of the hair loss experience. Some theorists believe that fear is at the root of all negative feelings — hence, conquering one's fears is crucial to a sense of belonging. Doing something pleasurable every day simply helps build positive feelings; the more pleasant feelings we enjoy on a daily basis, the fewer negative ones will be experienced. Tending to ones basic needs helps prevent unnecessary tension and discomfort, and enables one to feel less vulnerable to negative feelings about balding. Eating a balanced diet, exercising, getting a good nights rest are just a few of our basic human needs. Taking care of business means that you don't let the grueling little tasks of life get the best of you; it helps one feel more confident and competent. In comforting ourselves we learn that we don't have to rely on others for some of our physical needs. Along with enjoying a soak in a hot bath — or whatever one's choice for self-soothing might be — the realization that we can make a choice to be self-caring is empowering. Getting involved (or contributing) is a generous and loving way to distract ourselves from our own misery. The last (and most important) skill is to remember: You are not your hair. What's inside your head and in your heart is what truly matters.

CHAPTER EIGHT

THE LAST TANGLE

Resolving the Trauma of Hair Loss

A PROBLEM OR AN OPPORTUNITY?

Kate and Kathleen are identical twin sisters. At one time they looked almost exactly alike. They probably still do look alike, except for their hair. Several years ago Kate was in an automobile accident and after that her hair fell out. It never grew back in. Kate's doctors could not find a cause for her hair loss, so they said that it was emotional, probably due to the stress of the accident. Regardless of the cause, Kate went through a deeply painful and troublesome time. She wrote,

> *We get so caught up with fitting into an image that we forget who we are. I am more than just hair. So when I make television appearances and lecture around the country, my message is about overcoming obstacles. I talk to people about finding power in adversity, about turning tragedies into triumphs.*
> — Jojuan J. LaMorreaia

My hair loss has been a very tragic ordeal for me. I have a twin sister who has beautiful long hair — the way mine used to be — and I don't think I'll ever have that again. I went through some hiding times, and hating myself, and even punishing myself because I was so embarrassed at the way I looked. Wearing a wig was the toughest thing I ever had to do. People talked about me as if I had a terminal disease — and I didn't. But because I didn't know what it was [the cause of my hair loss] I really had nothing to say. Before I lost my hair I was very outgoing. But that changed completely. I became very quiet and shy.

Five years later I am still losing my hair, but I approach it in a different way. I am thankful for the hair I have. I have a loving family who really supports me, and I have an attitude about me in which I feel (and believe) that I can do anything. I know what I've gone through, and no one can take that experience away from me. Now I am a strong willed individual with a positive attitude on life — even if my hair is falling out!

Mourning the loss of one's hair can be an arduous process. Kate grieved the loss of her hair, and then moved on with her life. She began to appreciate what she had, rather than long for what she didn't have. She found inner strength, a strength that helped her view herself — and her life — more positively. And eventually she set new goals for herself. At the time of her writing she was in graduate school, working on a master's degree in counseling psychology.

Following the grief process there are many stages of adjustment to a personally threatening event, among them: (1) finding meaning in the event, (2) regaining control over the event and over one's life, and (3) feeling good about oneself again in spite of the personal setback.[1] Kate seems to have accomplished all three of these tasks. She eventually found value in her experience ("I know what I've gone through, and no one can take that away from me. Now I am a strong willed individual with a positive attitude on life"); she took charge of her life ("I have an attitude about me in which I feel, and believe, that I can do anything!"); she set new goals for herself (she was obtaining a graduate degree in her chosen field), a sign that she had reclaimed her sense of self-worth.

Finding Meaning in the Emotional Experience of Hair Loss

Traumatic events that affect an individual's personal life can be devastating, especially if the trauma involves a negative change in personal appearance. The face in the mirror is barely recognizable; friends, family members, even strangers, do not respond in the same way — a grim development, given that relationship support can go a long way in helping one cope.[2] What was once a predictable, orderly, understandable world is now an unfamiliar place. This can be shattering to an individual's sense of self in what now feels like a very different world, but sooner or later one tries to make sense of it all. Eventually the grieving individual tries to find a reason, generally spiritual, in the unfortunate event; a task that may be crucial to achieving a sense of well being. As Roxane Silver and Camille Wortman wrote, "psychological adjustment may well be influenced by the individual's ability to find meaning or purpose in his or her misfortune."[3]

For many individuals, identifying something positive in the experience of hair loss is the hardest task of all. It can be devastating, as losing one's hair is something that people will certainly notice. How can one possibly find something useful in the anguish of losing such a visible and distinctive part of the body? Mark said it was the first thing that people mentioned if they hadn't seen him in a while. When he returned to school in the fall of his senior year at Duke, his friends yelled, "Wow! You lost a lot of hair!!" He found this humiliating.

Finding something meaningful in the unwanted change of hair loss is a private, personal journey and, for some, a prolonged struggle. Several of the people that I spoke with had, however, resolved this first task. Roger was eventually able to view his hair loss as a humbling experience rather than a humiliating one. He said, "When I come across another person who is a balding male, I don't rag him about losing his hair. I am more sympathetic, because I understand. And it has also made me more aware of other issues, like people who are overweight or too tall." He was silent for a moment and added:

> At times I wonder, I mean, I say this jokingly ... but there is also a part of me that wonders about it. You know, is it my destiny? Did God select me for a lesson that I need to learn

"kind of thing?" It is a great lesson to learn. Sometimes I think that I wouldn't trade losing my hair for anything in the world.

Sheila supported Roger's feelings about being more understanding of others' physical flaws and misfortunes:

> I'm real sensitive to . . . not only to people like me . . . but to anybody with any kind of handicap. It really upsets me. I cannot stand to be around somebody and they're making a comment . . . I'll give 'em straight on that . . . about picking and saying little comments. It's hurtful! People can be so cruel . . . and say cruel, mean things.

Like Roger, Sheila alluded to a spiritual meaning in her hair loss when she said, "I believe that everything has a reason. I'm not real religious. I'm a Christian. But I believe that there was a reason for this. I don't know why, but there is a reason." Sheila's hair loss experience may have made her a better person. Her comment: "I believe it has."

Angela, who wants to become a nurse, spoke of a spiritual meaning she found in her experience of hair loss. She said:

> I do believe that something that is greater than me is giving me these experiences, so that when I become a care-giver again I will have total empathy with my patients. Not because I got it from a text book, but because I have lived it. I'd tell them that I'd been through it. And I would tell them that various other properties had made me different from the norm . . . that intelligence and beauty and dignity and love and compassion are all things that are within us. Hair loss is an outside thing. What we are . . . and what is important . . . is who we are inside.

Walt's discovery of meaning was more about personal growth:

> I think that going bald has really forced me to look at who I am and to either accept myself or reject myself, and I've accepted myself. And I think that if I had something [hair]

that made me more traditionally attractive to the opposite sex, I would probably get caught up in it and I'd become vain. I was very vain for a long time . . . especially when I was modeling. I felt like, "Well, you know, the world thinks I'm such a pretty person and, you know, and they're going to pay me all this money . . ."

He said that he would be "a lesser person" if he hadn't lost his hair . . . because he "would still be caught up in all that vain crap."

I used to be more superficial. I was much more vain. I was much more concerned with image. I really think that God has a plan for me, that is: You're going to learn these lessons . . . significantly.

Grace, you remember — lost her hair after a serious illness — talked about the solid bond she discovered in her marriage during this trying time.

Like the thing going on with my husband [he had been less affectionate while she was losing her hair] . . . we had just been through this incredible experience [her temporary paralysis] which was a very positive . . . in terms of our relationship . . . it was a real positive thing, in that he came through . . . big-time. And even though this [her hair loss] was happening . . . I didn't have major doubts, you know, about the relationship . . . or anything like that.

People who experience hair loss can feel helpless, even victimized. Finding a reason for this unwanted occurrence helps an individual bring meaning to the situation — and what it may symbolize about their existence on a deeper level. In other words, determining *why* it has occurred involves not only understanding the experience but also what the implications are for one's life in the present and future.

Human beings often feel the need to understand why a painful or traumatic event has occurred. Doing so brings stability to the situation. In addition, it helps them feel more secure in the world. For if an unfortunate event is understood, one might be able to prevent a similar occurrence in the future.[4] Regardless of how painful, enduring the search for significance (or meaning) can bring a different perspective on life and new knowledge about the self.[5]

Regaining Control Over One's Life

According to Shelley Taylor, a threatening event (such as hair loss) can easily undermine a person's sense of control over their body and over their life in general. People want "a feeling of control over the threatening event," said Taylor, "so as to manage it or [as mentioned] keep it from occurring again," a feeling that is exemplified by beliefs about personal control.[6]

Losing anything, including one's hair, can cause one to feel helpless — an overall, pervasive feeling of helplessness — and loss of control. Selena discussed this feeling.

> Maybe it has something to do with control. Because it's no problem if you have short hair if you cut it short, because you chose that! So maybe it's a 'you're not in control' kind of issue. It's something that is happening that you can't do anything about. It's very disturbing.

Yolanda said, "I really did feel a lot of despair associated with the fact that it was ... there were some things out of control. It was not within my control." She mentioned feeling helpless again when she said, "A part of me that I am supposed to have ... unless I choose to cut it off ... was gone ... leaving! I had no control over it."

The psychological stress that comes from loss of control is overwhelming, especially in the early stages of a potentially troubling event such as hair loss. The anticipatory stress — wondering if the loss will be ongoing and how much hair will fall out — can create severe anxiety and feelings of helplessness.[7] One way to challenge these feelings is to take control over the things that one has power over (change the things you can). "Stress reactions can be reduced," said Richard Lazarus, if the individual takes some form of action.[8] This can be accomplished by setting new and attainable, short term and long-term goals. Because hair loss can tamper with one's self-image, self-concept, and sexual esteem, an example of a goal would be to focus on new ways to be attractive and sensual.

The idea here is to develop an attitude about having control over as much of one's life as possible. Almost all of the people that I spoke with hadn't entirely given up on life, no matter how difficult it was. It was hard, but they took control and made purposeful decisions about everyday matters that helped them feel competent, confident, and in control. The idea is to be mindful about decision making. For example, Grace talked about how — in normal circumstances — hairstyles are something we can change (or have control over).

> I mean, how many times ... if you break up with a boyfriend, or whatever ... you go and change your hair. I might chose a perm, or get my hair frosted, or whatever. So when I went to rehab [for therapy following her stroke], I choose to get my hair cut.

This was a wise decision on Grace's part. Because the weight of longer, heavier hair pulls it close to the head (making it hug the scalp), shorter hair can actually camouflage the problem of thinning. A shorter style tends to make the hair spring upwards, giving it a fuller look."[9]

Selena spoke of taking control over the care of her rapidly thinning hair when she said,

> I did stop doing all kinds of stuff to my hair, because I felt that the curlers and the kinds of things I used to do to my hair would probably just be adding stress. I stopped curling my hair and any of the things I used to do to make my hair pretty ... anything that might "pull." I mean, washing my hair is a mess, because I take so much time and because it gets very tangled when it's wet. And I take ... just painstakingly ... because I'm trying to protect every single strand. I take a really long time, every time ... and I just use tons and tons of conditioners and try to keep as much hair on my head as possible.

Selena was also trying to protect her hair from the elements. She said that she purchased a cap to sleep in. "Not only to sleep in ... I wear it around the house all the time."

Helen took control of her hair loss in similar ways.

I don't use stuff on my hair. I don't spritz it. I don't mousse it. I don't apply heat to it. I only comb it, maybe once or twice a day. And I've only used a "pick" on it for almost 20 years. Because I don't want to accelerate the hair loss or do anything that's going to ... to exacerbate what I consider is already a problem.

And in an effort to provide her body (and hair) with proper nutrition:

I'm trying to stay as natural in my body maintenance as possible. And so ... you know, I try to not take drugs. I take vitamins and eat very little meat, and ... you know ... try and buy organic vegetables, and that kind of thing. And I've been eating like that for years, and I feel like it has done as right by me as anything could.

Helen is correct in believing that proper care of her body will help reduce the risk of further hair loss. Since food deprivation (or malnutrition)[10] can cause hair loss, it stands to reason that sufficient, balanced food intake can promote hair growth. Hair is a living organism and is vulnerable to the same forces (internal and external) that affect all other body parts. According to Neil Sadick and Donald Richardson, "The condition of a person's hair depends on his or her general health — both physical and mental — diet, and even the amount of sleep regularly gotten."[11] Certain vitamins have also been shown to be helpful. Vitamin A derivatives are reported to stimulate hair growth,[12] and one study indicated that cancer patients receiving Vitamin E supplements did not experience hair loss while on one specific chemotherapy.[13]

Hattie took control when she made a conscious decision about enduring painful treatments (steroid injections) for her hair loss. She first spoke about her sister, who was also experiencing hair loss: "She wouldn't like taking injections, 'cause she's scared of needles! I mean, I'm scared of 'em, too. But anything to help me, I'm for it. You know, that's the way I look at it." Hattie also made a decision about how to converse with her co-workers about her hair loss. When she was asked if she was on radiation, she said, "No, I have alopecia, which is a problem that causes hair loss. And I dropped it."

I just dropped it, and went off and left them standing there.

And I came back, and by that time they were sitting in their seats, you know. So, I felt that I didn't need to go into the details with them . . . what my problems were. So it was better that I just tell them what I had, and let them hang out there for a while.

Roger, too, made solid decisions about how (and how not) to style his thinning hair. He said that he would never wear a "flap" (an old-fashioned method to hide hair loss, whereby the hair is grown long on one side and combed over the top). He said that he had to find older female hairdressers who were willing to listen to him and try other ways of disguising his baldness. A flap . . . "rarely fools anyone," say Sadick and Richardson.

In reality, no hairstyle using only the remaining hairs on an individual's head can completely and naturally camouflage hair loss. However, making the best use of remaining hair is usually accomplished by curling and lifting the hair.[14]

Later, Roger declared a firm decision about another option: "I will never . . . so help me God! I will never use a toupee! I'm not going to do it."

Some men are in the mood for false hair, however. The improved techniques in making wigs and toupees (since the late 1950s) have led to a huge increase in the sale of men's hairpieces. And why not? Men are more conscious than ever about their hair loss. Furthermore, those handsome men on the screen have been wearing rugs and toupees for years.[15]

The task of setting goals as an effort to move beyond grief is generally easier to accomplish, as most people gain momentum when they begin thinking about changes they desire and have control over. Examples are: going back to school, changing a career, buying a house, losing weight, or taking a long-desired vacation. The focus is no longer on "what was" or "what is," but on "what can be." The individual is now looking more toward the future, rather than dwelling on the past.

A few of the people that I spoke with offered ways that they had (at some point) begun to take control and look to the future. After noticeable hair loss and a miserable first year in college, Dave set a goal of focusing on his classwork.

> I didn't know where I was going with my life. I knew I wanted to achieve something, but certainly wasn't doing it. My freshman grades were awful, and in large part because I didn't study or take it very seriously. No excuses there. And during my sophomore year I did better in school. And even though I was taking easy classes, I knew that when I signed up next year I could do very well. You know, in the major and in other classes. And I did!

Ralph said, "In spite of everything . . . not only have I achieved the goals, but I've surpassed them . . . always looking to go that extra yard. That's what makes me so successful at what I'm doing as far as market research."

Yolanda indicated a focus on the future when she spoke of her plans to take graduate courses during the summer months. Grace, too, indicated that she was leaving the past behind.

> I was real excited that I could . . . that I was able to go back to work. I kind of didn't want to, because of my baby. You know, 'cause I'd missed all that time with him. And then he was going to have to go into daycare right away. But I also knew that we needed the money . . . my husband had just started working on his own. I mean, all this happened at the same time . . . you know . . . I had the baby, the stroke, and my husband's boss that he'd been working with for five years was leaving to go to New Mexico. So, he was going to be on his own. And so . . . you know . . . I was thinking that I needed to go to work. I had to do that.

As mentioned, another way of taking control might involve a focus on one's personal appearance — which is difficult, because for the human species, hair has an appeal all of its own. More than anything, it seems to be a sexual thing. Perhaps not consciously, but it does seem to have something to do with feeling attractive to one's partner (or potential partner). We can understand why women feel this so strongly, but why men?

Since male pattern baldness is viewed as a sign of getting older, and because old age is generally accompanied by a loss of libido, a man might see his receding hairline as the first sign of an approaching impotence. Hence, a fear of balding (by men) is believed by some to be consistent with a fear of losing the ability to perform sexually — even though modern medicine has shown that balding has little or nothing to do with a loss of sexual prowess. Many women are actually attracted to balding males. Regardless, many men fear a loss of sexual attractiveness when they lose their hair.[16]

Hair *is* a sensual part of the human species, but it isn't the only sexual or sensual aspect of the human body. Eyes can be sensual — and the mouth, the legs, the buttocks, one's posture, and even one's attitude. There are other ways to be sensual and sexy besides owning a head of hair. Dave said that he was "taking the glasses off . . . and going back to contacts" in hopes of improving his appearance.

Angela looked for attractive ways to hide her baldness. She said that at first she tried a wig, but

after I got it, I wouldn't wear it, because it wasn't me. I mean, it just wasn't me at all. I eventually — during this period — went to a drugstore, and they had these kind of little "kerchief things" and I got several of those. And I liked those. They are very funky, and they were in style. They were cute. I've got some that I would probably wear right now.

She elaborated on this when she talked about helping other women who were experiencing baldness. "Get yourself a turban, baby . . . the wildest, craziest one you can find . . . and sew rhinestones on it!"

Roger was losing his hair before he was twenty years old, while he was still in college (on the coast of North Carolina).

What I did was get a tan as quickly as possible. And then I started dressing like a *surfer dude*. I'd wear baggy shorts, baggy shirts, and then I'd wear Ray-Ban sunglasses. And so I was able to fit into the crowd a little better.

And Helen, whose hair was thinning rapidly during adolescence, said that her mother bought her a fall (a shoulder-length hair piece).

It was like . . . you know . . . the glass slipper fitting. You know, it was just this transformed personal esteem of "Ahh! This is who I really could be." It gave me something that I didn't have naturally. It was almost like a superhuman kind of feeling . . . like the Wonder Woman kind of thing. It was that kind of . . . when Wonder Woman puts on her special belt.

As Helen got older she found that having female idols (or role models) who were less concerned about their appearance — and more interested in their achievements — very helpful.

I took on my crone images from women like Georgia O'Keeffe. I don't recall seeing too many pictures of her after the 30s . . . where her hair is actually showing, but this type of woman is . . . to me . . . represents women who are secure in their crone years, and are not concerned about whether they have scalp hair or not. Because they just always wore hats. I'm definitely . . . this is a head for hats . . . and, you know, I love hats. They're not terribly . . . not always practical . . . but certainly, as a Senior citizen, I feel like I could get away with wearing as many hats as I wanted . . . all the time . . . because I love hats. And, they wore hats, and it was okay with them.

Renata Polt said that she purchased three wigs, each styled differently, but that she wore each one only a few times, because all of them were scratchy . . . "once my head had been reduced to bare scalp."

So what did I wear? I started with scarves. When I wanted to feel dressed-up, I wound a large cotton scarf around my head, adapting the styles of Black Muslim women I studied on the street. Later, I acquired a few caps, the most useful of which was a multicolored cotton crochet number of the sort once favored by Whoopi Goldberg. It was floppy and unflattering, but it was comfortable and went with just about everything.[17]

Melissa, however, shared a different and interesting point of view.

There was this lady that my aunt saw on TV that . . . it was a couple of years ago, I think. This lady is a black lady, and all of her hair is shaved off. And she shaved her eyebrows also, and used an eyebrow pencil. She wears a lot of makeup and fancy earrings, and my aunt said she was really pretty the way she looked. I don't remember why her hair fell out . . . if she had alopecia or what . . . but my aunt said she looked pretty like that, and she told me that maybe I should try that.

That lady might have been Jojuan LaMorreaia, an African American female who lost all of her hair — including brows and lashes — in 1977, to alopecia. Jojuan is now a motivational speaker and the founder of the Center for Self-Esteem and the National Alopecia Network. Both organizations are located in Detroit.[18]

There is help, however, for those individuals who do not want to go bareheaded. In most cities there is at least one individual (generally, a female) who advertises assistance with makeup, wig selection, and how to create a pleasing image when bald (or balding). This individual is usually found through a local hospital or beauty salon. To my knowledge there is no current title for this career. I would suggest *cosmetherapist*.

Increasing Self-Esteem

Self-esteem is an elusive and complex human quality. Simply stated, it is the relationship that an individual has with him — or herself, friendly or unfriendly. It develops over time, and can change at any given moment — depending on the experiences that we have and how we handle them. Having good self-esteem requires

1. a reasonably strong sense of *self* (and one's values) — and being true to that self — while showing respect, regard, and concern for others,

2. acknowledging and handling the difficult problems (and subsequent choices) in life; and

3. accepting life on life's terms, such as adjusting to all of the losses that sooner or later come to all of us.

Self-esteem has a lot to do with knowing and accepting oneself as an imperfect being, appreciating one's positive traits, and trying to improve on the negative ones. Self-esteem does not come from an outside source. Attaining good self-esteem is the result of *inner* work, yet is often visible to the *outer* world. It is a lonely, but rewarding journey.

When an individual is losing (or has lost) his or her hair, an important part of his — or her uniqueness is affected. It undermines one's selfhood, or how one perceives him — or herself in the world. As was evident with almost all of the people I spoke with, and as Dalma Heyn wrote, "Hair has a powerful effect on our moods and identity."[19]

> Anyone who has watched her hair break off by the handful after too much processing (several of you) or fall out mysteriously during or after pregnancy (several more of you) or leave the scalp in clumps as a result of disease (just a few of you) knows about revenge, and about the cost of such betrayal to the psyche.[20]

The wound to the psyche is true for men as well as women. Bret said that losing his hair at a very young age made him feel uncomfortable. He said that he didn't fit in with his crowd: "In situations like being in a class full of other people ... you know ... it would tend to make me a little quieter or a little more self-conscious than I normally would have been . . . just the feeling of being different and, therefore, people are looking at you." Jake, who also lost his hair while a college student, said, "It's tough to try to speak up in a crowd when all of a sudden everyone looks at you, and you know that they're categorizing you physically . . . especially when it's a room full of strangers."

An improvement in self-esteem was evident in several of the individuals that I spoke with — but only with men — and more often than not, it was consistent with having a successful, significant relationship. Walt, who was twenty-six years old at the time of our meeting, said that he was more comfortable with himself now than he was when he was twenty and first losing his hair. "Not that I like everything about myself, but I'm better able to deal with accepting what I don't like and changing it, without having to beat myself up to do it." Later in the interview, Walt added, "What's real is that your wife loves you for who you are, and so . . . I think, for me, it's been a way for me to learn that there's something more important than the way you look."

At the end of his interview, Bret indicated an improvement in his self-esteem when he said,

> I deal with it [hair loss] a lot better than I used to. I don't know, I dealt with it okay, I guess. [But] the situation was different before I was married. And you know, ten years ago, or whatever, going out to bars with your friends and everything, your priorities and your orientations are different.

Dave, too, seemed to be gaining a brighter perspective on the issue of physical appeal and hair loss. He said, "It bothered me less and less as time went on . . . which is still true. It bothers me very little now. As my self-esteem turned around, the hair became less important very rapidly." He then decided that his baldness could give him a little *class*.

Roger indicated an increase in self-esteem when he talked about the jokes made about balding men. He said, "I used to be embarrassed. But now I begin to think, 'What is it about *you* that is making *you* tell this joke . . . so that *you* feel good about yourself . . . and in doing that you are putting me down?' It used to be . . . 'Gee . . . I feel pretty badly about myself!' But not so much anymore."

It was a different story for women, however. Few of the females that I interviewed had reached a point of feeling better about themselves after losing their hair. Yolanda came close when she said,

> So, if my hair came back . . . it would be . . . like the culmination of . . . of finally getting it all back together. Because everything really is great. I have a great job, the kids are doing great, my husband is paying child support . . . you know, financially things are really okay I've started dating . . . actually dating . . . and feeling comfortable about dating. So, if I . . . were to have hair, it would be like the final thing of all. I mean, I'm not going to get my marriage back. You know, I mean, that's a loss . . . and I've dealt with it.

Melissa, however, represented what most of the women felt:

My self-esteem has been really low. And I kind of shy away from certain situations. Like even with wearing a wig, there are things that happen. Like it seems like when I start to get really comfortable with it, it will be a windy day like it is outside now, and my wig will blow off. I think that I would have better self-esteem if I had hair. I would say, that if I had hair like everybody else, I don't even think that if I had long hair . . . or a good texture hair . . . if I just had hair! You know, if I had a head full of hair . . . there are lots of ways you can style your hair and make yourself look good.

Women, not surprisingly, expressed lower self-esteem (and greater emotional distress) over losing their hair than men. This was validated in the results of the "Feelings About Hair Loss Question-naire"[21] and was not a shocking revelation, given that women in our society feel pressured to define themselves through their physical appearance. It seems that a woman's self-esteem is closely connected to her ability to look pretty — along with the fact that there are differences in males' and females' self-esteem in general. "Men," wrote Freedman, "generally start from a stronger position," meaning that women have difficulty competing with men in many areas. The one area in which men cannot compete with women is in feminine beauty and charm. To a woman, then, losing hair can mean more than a loss of self-worth. It can mean a loss of secret strength, personal power, and finesse.[22]

According to Freedman, the inner image of a woman's body is so closely connected with self-esteem that "distortion of one literally deforms the other." If a woman fails to retain her attractiveness, she begins to feel helpless "with regard to controlling a fundamental aspect" of her feminine identity. The sad truth is that women — unlike men — are often judged by things over which they have no control.[23]

Regardless, low self-esteem as a result of hair loss is present for men as well as women. Many of the men that I spoke with said that they, too, are affected by the forces of physical attractiveness, indicating that women are not the only ones held to standards of beauty.

Research has shown that first impressions of bald men are generally ranked lower (than their hair-gifted peers) on many levels: physical attractiveness, life success, social attractiveness, self-assertiveness, intelligence, personal likability, and estimation of age.[24] According to Tom Cash, "baldness is viewed negatively by the general public."

> Research has shown that balding men are sometimes judged to be five years older than their actual age and thought to be less assertive in business and personal relationships, less successful, even less likable.[25]

Roger said, "It's definitely apparent to me in the business world that image is very important. I mean we are constantly bombarded with commercials on TV about the way we look. And so, I am definitely aware and wondering what other people think of me, and my image. Do they like me because I look a certain way? Mostly, I think about how I will be perceived in comparison to other people. You know, how many times do you see a young, bald male as a sexy model?"

"In our society, hair styles and the importance of having hair are encouraged through the media," said Walt.

> They pound it into you, "this is how you're supposed to look." And you're supposed to be cool, and you're supposed to be suave, and it's normal for women to fawn over you. And you're supposed to look like all the guys on soap operas. It's just like women who get bombarded with images of Playboy bunnies and that sort of thing. It really is a traumatic thing.

"Like in *Seinfeld* a couple of weeks ago," said Mark, "that was a big thing about getting the hair piece and stuff. And that was funny. I mean, you know, I can't say that wasn't funny. I mean, you know, look how George is depicted: the short, fat, bald guy."

What these men are telling us is that hair is one of the assets that helps them feel either included (in society) or excluded. Walt, Mark, and Roger — all experiencing male pattern baldness — indicated that they felt judged or perceived in ways that were not attractive.

Because hair is vital to one's personal identity, its' loss is likely to have emotional consequences for anyone experiencing hair loss — male or female. As evidenced by all of the people I spoke with, experiencing hair loss can take its toll on one's self-regard.

Restructuring One's Life Around Hair Loss

We live in a society that values physical attractiveness. It is relentless, and at times unforgiving. This social environment, coupled with the anguish of losing a truly visible and quite personal part of the body, makes it difficult for an individual to resolve painful feelings about hair loss. Hair is important — not only to the social self — but to the sexual and cultural self. Hair is important to one's being, and to lose it can be devastating. In the end, however, suffering such a loss can be an opportunity to mature and change. One can grow because of it (as Kate did). It can make one psychologically richer and emotionally stronger.[26] To get mired in painful feelings about something over which one has no control can only result in an uneasy life. As Victor Frankl said, "As long as we are still suffering from a condition that ought not to be, we remain in a state of tension between what actually is on the one hand and what ought to be on the other hand."[27]

Human beings are an amazing species, however. Human beings can adjust. They can find meaning in unpleasant events, set new life courses, and create illusions to help them cope with painful losses. Shelley Taylor said:

> My biologist acquaintances frequently note that the more they know about the human body the more, not less, miraculous it seems. The recuperative powers of the mind merit similar awe. The process of cognitive adaptation [using one's mental processes to control one's emotions, perceptions, motivations, and behaviors] to threat, though often time-consuming and not always successful, nonetheless restores many people to their prior level of functioning and inspires others to find new meaning in their lives. For this reason, cognitive adaptation occupies a special place in the roster of human capabilities.[28]

Losing one's hair can be a traumatic and emotionally troubling experience for all of the reasons mentioned in this book. It is a loss that some people never resolve. Many do!

Resolving the emotional experience of hair loss is an exercise in *adaptation*. It begs a reshaping of values about how one perceives him — or herself in the mirror and in the world. In a society that bombards us with attractive images of human beauty and perfection, this period of adjustment asks that we go a little deeper, that we examine our perceptions of ourselves, and adjust our concept of self. This takes time.

The processes around which *adaptation* occur include (1) finding meaning in the emotional experience of hair loss, (2) regaining control over this unwanted change (and one's life), and (3) improving one's self-esteem. Finding significance in the experience of hair loss involves looking beyond the possible cause and determining how one can use the setback for future good. Gaining mastery (or control) requires a *take-charge* attitude over the things in life that we do have control over (which might include the purchase of hair growth products). An unwanted experience like hair loss can easily threaten a person's feelings of control over their body and over their life. Hence, part of the adjustment to losing one's hair involves gaining a sense of personal control (or mastery) over as much of one's life as possible. Enhancing one's self-esteem requires understanding the nature of self-esteem and getting to work on developing a healthy relationship with the *self*.

CHAPTER NINE

MYTH, MAGIC, AND MEDICINE

Past, Present, and Future Treatments for the Regrowth of Hair

DOG'S TOES, HORSES' TEETH, AND BLACK LIZARDS

Throughout history people have tried numerous interesting (and sometimes vile) concoctions in attempts to regrow their lost hair. The first such reported remedy — a topical application, one hopes — was prepared nearly 5,000 years ago and was developed for a woman, the queen of Egypt:

> Hairs may be transplanted, and it is said, will grow after such transplantation, in consequence of the adhesions and organic connection established between them and the adjacent tissues; a fact, of which practical advantage might be taken, if correct.
> — Dr. Arthur Hill Hassell (1817-1894)

Ses, Mother of His Majesty, the king of Upper and Lower Egypt. It was composed of the "Toes-of-a-Dog, Refuse-of-Dates, Hoof-of-an-Ass."[1] Another recorded Egyptian practice used to stimulate hair growth was to soak the tooth of an ass in honey and rub it on the scalp. The most foul and disgusting preparations that the balding Egyptians ever doused on their scalps, however, must be either "Vulva, Phallus, and the Black Lizard," or "Writing fluid, Fat-of-the-Hippopotamus, and Gazelle's dung."[2]

There are no reports available recounting success (or failure) when using these outrageous methods, but given such efforts, one can only imagine that the people of this ancient civilization struggled as much with the social and psychological implications of hair loss as do people today. Fortunately their treatments became less repulsive, as a later method reported to have been used was a type of witchcraft (or exorcism) involving the sun's rays:

To Charm Away Alopecia

O Shining One, Thou who hoverest above!
O Xare! O Disc of the Sun!
O Protector of the Divine Neb-apt!

To be spoken over

Iron
Red-lead
Onions
Alabaster
Honey
Make into one and give against.[3]
[Mixed and applied to the scalp?]

By the mid-1800s there were fewer such remedies around to cure hair loss and a greater focus on cause and prevention. Alexander Rowland said that "fall of the hair" may be a result of worry and stress, a "disorder of the digestive organs," overeating, or an infection on the scalp. He identified "the sun's rays" as a possible cause of baldness, along with the "fumes of quicksilver," wearing a "military cap or helmet," and the use of tobacco. For treatment he suggested "frequent cutting" of the hair and proper attention to the gastrointestinal tract (as well as the entire body).[4]

Rowland also blamed "contraction or relaxation" of the scalp as a cause of baldness, and he suggested a way that might reverse the problem — one that increased circulation to the hair follicles:

Strong local irritation, producing a tendency of blood to the part, has frequently been found efficacious in restoring the hair in bald places on the head. Blistering; the application of caustic potash; and an ointment composed of cantharides and lard, have been severally tried, with more or less advantage.[5]

One of the more interesting ideas Rowland presented was a presumed cause of baldness in men — and women, if they were sufficiently gifted. He said that men who overexerted "their intellectual powers" (i.e., scientists, theologians, accountants) were more likely to lose their hair. Women — should they be even minimally inclined to use their brains — would also be vulnerable to hair loss and should cover this affliction:

> The hair of men more commonly falls off than that of women; and they become bald from the greater excitement of the brain which their pursuits occasion. Bald women are scarcely ever seen; nevertheless, some ladies who follow the pursuits of literature are obliged to cover their baldness with head dresses of hair prepared by the coiffeur.[6]

By the late 1800s, new and varied explanations and treatments for hair loss were emerging. Dr. Henri Leonard identified possible causes to be syphilis, high fever, nerve injuries (such as psychological shock), irregular bowel movements, problems with the uterus, the excessive use of tobacco, wearing a hat, and "a gradual failing of the systemic powers" (perhaps referring to the aging process).[7] Tonics, lotions, and pomades for the scalp were recommended for treatment, along with adequate sleep, exercise, general relaxation, and a reduction in smoking. He said that the "bowels should be kept regular," and he recommended several laxative preparations — among them a mixture of cascara sagrada, buckthorn bark, simple syrup, and cinnamon water, to be taken as one "dessertspoonful before breakfast, or three times a day if necessary."[8]

Leonard recommended that the scalp be kept as clean as possible, and he advised the application of several tonics, most of them containing Spanish fly, some type of oil (sweet almond or castor) and cologne water. He also mentioned "a preparation of arsenic, given internally," and cautioned that it should not be "prescribed indiscriminately."[9]

Leonard agreed with Rowland that an increased blood flow to

the scalp could stimulate the regrowth of hair, but his suggestion for treatment was a bit more radical:

> Electricity applied, with proper care, to the scalp by means of a wet sponge, one of the poles of the battery being placed at the nape of the neck, will also be found of service in stimulating the nervous action, and thus increase the amount of blood sent to each hair follicle and its papilla.[10]

By the mid-1900s, newer, more tolerable remedies were emerging that proclaimed to cure baldness, and progress was being made toward understanding the causes of hair loss. Certain illnesses were considered prime offenders, especially those that were accompanied by a high fever.[11] Heredity and hormonal imbalances[12] were also being linked to hair loss. Yet other causes were suggested that would not hold up today: eye strain, a nervous disposition, germs, and dandruff.[13] Drs. Oscar Levin and Howard Behrman said that nine out of ten patients who sought treatment for baldness suffered from dandruff. They also blamed "micro-organisms or parasites" and suggested that such varmints were spread by "infected combs, brushes, towels, and hats." The physical ailments mentioned as possible causes of hair loss were: "stomach troubles, disorders of the intestines, and derangements of the endocrines."[14] Levin and Behrman wrote:

> Acidosis and autointoxication, the results of faulty diet and elimination, are revealed in tests of the blood and urine of seemingly healthy patients who apply for treatment of premature baldness. Persons with good constitutions may suffer, in other words, but those with weak constitutions are more apt to suffer, and suffer worse, from premature baldness.[15]

The prescribed treatment for hair loss at this time (by Levin and Behrman) involved:

- The proper care and treatment of the whole body.
- Thorough and continual cleansing of the affected area.
- Removing the scales, scabs and crusts.
- Killing the germs of infection.

- Soothing the inflamed tissues.
- Applying drugs which act on the glands of the scalp.[16]

If heredity were believed to be the cause of an individual's hair loss, Levin and Behrman recommended impeccable cleanliness and daily scalp massage:

> With this massage the scalp should be pinched and pulled up. This loosens the fat tissue and the fibers and helps keep them flexible and lively, and improves the circulation. Vibration is also of benefit. If the scalp is dry it should be rubbed daily with one of the bland oils already mentioned [almond, olive, cod liver].[17]

Vitamins were also suggested as possible cures for baldness, possibly due to the fact that certain vitamin deficiencies were known to cause hair loss. Levin and Behrman recommended vitamins A, C, D, E, K, P (found in vitamin C and known as "citrin") and a combination of B vitamins. They also identified the use of penicillin and sulfa drugs — perhaps the only antibiotics available at that time — as helpful against scalp infections and subsequently against hair loss.[18]

Treatment of Hair Loss and the Advancement of Medical Science

We know today that systemic conditions (i.e., malnutrition, anemia, hormonal imbalances) can and do cause hair loss, and all should be ruled out before treatment begins. Heredity can also be a factor. This means that when seeking medical help for hair loss, a complete family and medical history is in order, along with a total physical examination.[19] Rodney Dawber and Dr. Dominique Van Neste say that, in their experience, "up to ten percent of those who complained of hair loss were diagnosed as suffering from hypothyroidism [underactive thyroid function]." The patients were subsequently treated with thyroid hormones, and their hair growth was restored to normal within eight weeks.[20] Psychological stress can also be a factor in hair loss,[21] along with the use of certain medications (i.e., oral contraceptives); these causes, too, must be ruled out.[22] Occasionally the cause of an individual's hair loss is simply unknown; when a physician is unable to determine the cause, the patient's disposition is, sadly, sometimes blamed.[23]

Current diagnostic terms indicating some of the common and uncommon causes of hair loss are as follows:

- **Alopecia areata** is a term that simply denotes hair loss. A. Jarrett, E. Johnson, and R. Spearman say that alopecia areata is a "relatively common condition, but has no proven genetic control, although there is evidence of positive family histories." They say that some cases appear to be caused by stress, but the actual cause (to date) is unknown.[24] Dr. Maria Hordinsky gives a physiological explanation, stating that with this condition a high degree of inflammation has been noted around the hair follicle, that it weakens and the hair breaks off.[25]

- **Trichorrhexis Nodosa** refers to hair loss caused by overtreatment, such as frequent shampooing with harsh cleansing agents or prolonged and intense brushing. These treatments cause the hair to lose its normal moisture, become unusually brittle, and break. Trichorrhexis nodosa can be caused by using permanent waving lotions and hydrogen peroxide (to lighten the hair).[26]

- **Androgenic alopecia** refers to male pattern baldness. U. Schumacher-Stock says that it comes about as a result of an "endogenous increase in androgen level, administration of androgens, increased susceptibility of hair follicles to androgenic stimuli."[27] H. Baden notes, however, that the blood levels of other male hormones, such as testosterone, do not appear to change "between balding and non-balding individuals."[28] The cause of female pattern alopecia is also believed to be androgen related, but Baden says that it is "modified in its presentation by female genetic factors."[29] Ninety-five percent of androgenic alopecia is believed to be linked to hereditary factors.[30]

- **Telogen Effluvium** refers to hair loss following periods of stress, a serious illness, or pregnancy. Dawber and Van Neste say that "fever, prolonged and difficult childbirth, surgical operations, hemorrhage (including blood donation), sudden severe reduction of food intake ('crash dieting') and emotional stress, including perhaps that of prolonged jet flights," may all contribute to this type of hair loss.[31]

- **Trichotillomania** is a type of alopecia that results from repeated and deliberate hair plucking. According to Dawber and Van Neste, this behavior "occurs more than twice as frequently in females as in males," is more common in children than in adults, and is at times an unconscious act.[32] Trichotillomania is a psychological condition that is difficult to treat.

- **Scarring**: Accident or injury to the scalp can be severe enough to destroy hair follicles and result in baldness to the affected site. People have been known to be scalped in automobile accidents, resulting in destruction of the hair follicles; burns and topical drugs (i.e., para-amino salicylic acid or quinacrine) can also cause scarring and subsequent hair loss.[33]

- **Drug-induced hair loss**: a cause of hair loss that is becoming more common as newer and more powerful medications are introduced to the market. Types of drugs that could potentially cause one's hair to fall out are: birth control pills, antihypertensive medications, amphetamines, androgens, anticoagulants, anticholesterol preparations, as well as high doses of aspirin. Drugs used in chemotherapy treatments are almost guaranteed to cause hair loss because they attack the fastest-growing cells in the body (cancer cells as well as hair follicles).[34]

- **Hypothyroidism** refers to a deficiency in the activity of the thyroid gland (insufficient secretion of the thyroid hormone). It is a condition that may cause significant hair loss.[35]

- **Trauma**, such as pulling the hair back tightly, braiding (especially cornrows), even wearing a tight wig can cause one's hair to thin (or break).[36]

Currently, there are four types of treatment available to replace or encourage the regrowth of hair: surgical procedures, steroid injections, topical applications, and oral medication. The treatment of choice for optimal results must be tailored to a proper diagnosis,[37] says Dr. Maria Hordinsky. As mentioned earlier, a thorough medical examination, a solid medical history, and sometimes a psychological evaluation are required before treatment begins.

HAIR RESTORATION — SURGICAL PROCEDURES

"The primary goal of many hair replacement surgeons," say Drs. Kenneth Buchwach and Raymond Konior, "is to remove as much of a patient's bald area as possible."[38] This can be done by moving small plugs of hair from one section to another (*hair transplantation*[39]) or by stretching the scalp (*scalp reduction*[40]), lifting it (*scalp lift*[41]), or rotating it to another area (*scalp flap*[42]). A part-surgical/part-cosmetic procedure that can also create a new head of hair is the *implant*.[43] The choice for one surgery (or procedure) over another is made through the advice of a plastic surgeon, as not all individuals seeking surgical restoration of their hair are appropriate candidates for all available procedures.

Punch Graft Hair Transplantation

A hair transplant involves the grafting of small chunks of hair from active sites on the patient's scalp to the balding area.[44] The small grafts of hairy scalp — commonly referred to as *donor grafts* or *plugs* — are placed into recipient holes on the balding scalp that have been made smaller than those used to obtain the donor grafts. The reason for the smaller recipient site, says Dr. Walter Unger, is that plugs, or grafts, "tend to 'shrink' somewhat after they are removed from the donor site and recipient holes tend to slightly enlarge."[45] Hair transplantation is an involved and time-consuming project for the patient. There is an evaluation period, a planning phase, a series of surgical transplants, and a short recovery period following each procedure (both the donor sites and the recipient sites must heal). The number of transplant surgeries depends, of course, on the degree of baldness presented and the amount of hair desired by the patient.

Two common reasons for candidates being rejected for hair transplant are an insufficient supply of adequate donor sites (not enough hair left to transplant to another site) and a hair loss pattern of all-over thinning. Women often fall into the pervasive thinning pattern, or low-density hair growth, mainly due to the diffuse character of hair loss commonly experienced with female pattern baldness.[46]

Complications can result from this type of surgery — as with any invasive medical procedure — such as infection, excessive bleeding, pruritus (intense itching), swelling, or donor site problems such as a "pluggy" (or tufted) appearance.[47] It goes without saying that all risks and possible complications should be discussed with one's surgeon during the consultation and planning phase of treatment.

Scalp (Alopecia) Reduction

Scalp reduction is the surgical removal of portions of bald skin on the scalp, with the remaining scalp (that is bearing hair) stretched to cover the excision. As with a hair transplant, the number of surgeries required depends on the amount of skin to be excised, along with the patient's desired outcome. This surgery seems to be a relatively simple and predominantly successful procedure, but according to Dr. James Swinehart, it can be somewhat tricky — especially when deciding how to cover the excised area or how to expand the hair-bearing scalp. Regardless, there are a variety of surgical maneuvers that can accomplish the task,[48] such as the use of an expander, a balloon-type device inserted beneath the hair-bearing skin, slowly stretching it. The use of this device also allows for removal of more bald skin per session.[49] Another option for covering the excised part is to use a flap (moving a strand of hair-bearing scalp to the area).[50] Some say that a scalp reduction performed in combination with a hair transplant can also achieve a desirable outcome.[51]

A scalp reduction works best for patients who have a lot of scalp to give, in other words, they have sufficient skin elasticity. Drs. Toby Mayer and Richard Fleming say that the patient with a tight scalp is simply not a good candidate for the procedure, "since the amount of gain usually does not justify the resulting scar, nor the time and expense."[52]

Complications generally associated with scalp reduction are (1) stretch-back, (2) scarring, (3) loss of hair around the suture line, and (4) continued hair loss, requiring more surgery in the future.[53] Sometimes the tissue that has been stretched wants to reexpand (stretch-back); however the use of newer techniques (i.e., the expander) are reported to successfully reduce this complication.[54] Scars (which can be wide, depressed, and quite visible[55]) and loss of hair around the incision can also be problems — two complications that, according to the experts, can be minimized significantly with transplant procedures.[56] Intense pain and infection can be immediate postsurgical problems, but both can be handled adequately with appropriate medication.[57] The problem of continued hair loss can also be a complication following a scalp reduction (or, for that matter, following any hair restoration procedure). The chance of experiencing this complication would depend, of course, on the origin of the patient's hair loss.

Scalp Lift

A scalp lift is basically an improvement on standard reduction, one difference being that it allows the surgeon to excise more bald skin. As with a reduction, surgical incisions are made on the scalp, the bald area is excised, and the sides are brought together and sutured. Only two procedures are required, however, when choosing this type of hair restoration surgery: the *bilateral* scalp lift is done first, followed with the *bitemporal* scalp lift. When undergoing the bilateral lift, the incision looks much like a horseshoe (laying flat), with the long lines extending from the crown to the temporal areas.[58] The bitemporal scalp lift follows the bilateral lift by three or more months, with most of the scarring from the previous surgery being excised in the process. Once again the sides are brought together, and the excised region is covered with the patient's own hair. When the surgical sites are healed, the crown is given hair with the help of three or four transplant sessions.[59]

Possible complications that can result from a scalp lift are (1) tissue necrosis — an eroding of scalp tissue — due to lack of blood flow to the surgical site, (2) loss of hair around the suture line (already discussed), (3) infection, and (4) numbness. A prescribed regimen of preoperative antibiotics can prevent the development of an infection. Numbness, however, can be a temporary (lasting a few months) or even permanent situation.[60]

Scalp Flap

Swinehart says that "the two proven surgical techniques for hair replacement are multiple graft techniques [transplant procedures] and scalp flap procedures," with scalp flap being his choice for optimal results. In his opinion, a scalp flap provides a more "natural and pleasing result as well as a more rapid completion."[61] A scalp flap requires excising a piece of hairbearing scalp and relocating it to a bald area. It can be performed in a variety of ways. One design uses patches of hair from the sides of the head and moves them to the front (Juri flap); another uses patches from the back and sides of the head and moves them to the front or top of the head (TPO, or temporal-parietal-occipital flap).[62] Surgeons are generally eager to make improvements on existing methods, and Mayer and Fleming did just that. They use a modified Juri flap (the Mayer-Fleming flap) and a modified inferiorly based temporoparietal flap; they state that these are better designs.[63] A variety of flap designs are used (and described) by leaders in the field.[64]

According to Sadick and Richardson, careful patient selection is the key to success with a scalp flap. They say that the best candidate for this surgery "has only frontal baldness with dark, coarse hairs behind." With this presentation, the flap will not only blend well into the existing hair, but will cover the bald area completely. Otherwise, the scalp flap can sit alone on top of the head, like an island of hair.[65]

Unger says that the primary advantage of flaps is that "when they are properly carried out they produce dense bands of hair growth," like a full head of hair. Furthermore, the results are almost always immediate and ongoing. Cosmetic disadvantages can occur, however — one being that the hair will grow in narrow bands and sometimes in different directions. Hence, styling the hair could be more of a problem.[66]

Possible complications of a scalp flap are scarring, especially in the donor section; necrosis (death of tissue); bleeding; and swelling. Scarring can also occur around the eroding (or necrotic) tissue, and can be minimized with a transplant procedure. One can expect a lengthy recovery period — as long as seven weeks — following this particular surgery, and the patient would need to prepare for this.[67]

The Implant

An implant is a relatively minor procedure whereby suture material is sewn directly into the scalp and a hair piece (i.e., wig) is attached to the sutures. The patient's own hair is then pulled through the net — the web of netting that holds the hair piece together — and is blended into the false hair, giving it a more natural appearance. The hair piece is generally uncut and unstyled at the time of the procedure, and is later trimmed and styled to suit the patient. Another type of implant involves multiple scalp sutures, with strands of false hair threaded in and through the stitches.[68] The false hair is then blended into the patient's natural hair. As simple and quickly rewarding as this procedure sounds, Sadick and Richardson are not in favor of implants (at the present time):

> The drawbacks to implants are similar to the general problems of wearing a wig except they are more severe. The sweating, oiliness, and cleanliness difficulties can all be present. Implants have fallen out of favor because of problems with severe infections and scarring as well as foreign-body reactions, which can be life-threatening.[69]

What's in the Future?

In regard to hair restoration surgery, what can we expect in the near future? "Hair follicle replication, or cloning," states Dr. Swinehart. He says that recent research has shown that one may not need the bulb region of the follicle to stimulate new hair growth, that other follicular components are capable of regenerating hair. He says that we're "a long way from generating an incubator full of hair," but it appears to be a promising technique for the future.[70]

According to Unger, two advances in hair restoration surgery are "the use of strip harvesting for the donor area and the development and perfection of the use of smaller grafts." One advantage with the harvesting technique is that it produces thinner (and fewer) scars in the donor supply area (allowing for greater use of donor tissue). The improvement in smaller grafts, he says, minimizes the "pluggy" appearance that comes with larger grafts. Another promising new development, writes Unger, "is the use of lasers for preparing recipient sites for smaller grafts." [71]

Points to Ponder

When considering hair restoration surgery, it is important to interview several plastic surgeons before making a final decision about who will do the work. When the choice for a surgeon is made, several appointments will be scheduled to discuss and plan the surgical process. However, before signing the consent forms and committing to the surgical process, there are several important issues to consider: (1) the long term effects of hair restoration surgery, (2) the cost, (3) the discomfort, and (4) the possibility of postsurgical complications.

If one is experiencing ongoing hair loss, chances are that it will continue after the surgery. Buchwach and Konior say that "most hair restoration procedures have been designed to treat the patient for the moment, without serious regard for their ultimate long-term effects on that patient."[72] This means that the final results of a surgical procedure (especially for a young patient) may not be recognized for several years.

Cost is another issue to consider. Ten years ago the cost of a scalp reduction was approximately $5,000. Today it is guaranteed to be higher. A transplant can range anywhere from $2,000 to $15,000, as the actual cost depends on the number of donor grafts needed to achieve the patient's desired aesthetic effect.[73] Weighing the cost with one's hopes and expectations is important. As mentioned above, the results of one's costly investment, regrettably, may not last long.

Surgical procedures invade the body. An individual undergoing hair restoration surgery may experience postoperative pain — or at the very least, discomfort — and may be in for a long convalescent period. There are, of course, ways to ameliorate physical discomfort (i.e., pain medication) and those means will certainly be provided. Regardless, it's important to know that it may take several days (maybe longer) before one can comfortably tolerate the aftermath of the procedure.

The most common complications that can result from hair restoration procedures have been identified, and those unpleasant possibilities should be discussed with the surgeon during the planning phase of treatment. Surgical complications are unexpected, but realistically they can occur. And when they do, further pain and discomfort, further expense, and sometimes additional surgery is necessary.

The Use of Intralesional Steroids in the Treatment of Hair Loss

Steroid injections are often used to treat alopecia areata, "particularly localized patches of alopecia areata," writes Hordinsky. The injections are administered directly into the patchy bald area(s) every one to two weeks, and if the treatment is satisfactory one might see the beginnings of hair regrowth as early as two weeks. Reports are favorable for using intralesional steroidal injections as long as (1) the patient presents with more than 50% of his or her scalp hair, (2) the progression of hair loss is slow to moderate, and (3) the duration of loss is less than two years.[74]

The drawbacks of using steroid injections are pain on administration and the possibility of atrophy (the wasting away of tissue in the site). The pain factor isn't a surprise, as most people anticipate discomfort when receiving injections in the scalp. Atrophy, however, is an unpleasant possibility to consider. Hordinsky says that "if injections are given too frequently and if atrophied areas are reinjected, the atrophy may become permanent and interfere with hair regrowth."[75]

The administration of intralesional and topical steroids have both been shown to be effective in the regrowth of hair, with intralesional steroid injections producing better results (especially in the management of small patches of alopecia,[76] which was the case with Hattie). The use of topical steroids has produced good results, but reports of success appear to center around patients whose hair growth could have occurred spontaneously (without any treatment).

Topical Applications that Encourage the Regrowth of Hair

Topical solutions are primarily used for alopecia areata. The most common types used are: (1) the hair follicle stimulant minoxidil; (2) sensitizing agents, such as dinitrochlorobenzene (DNCB), squaric acid dibutyl ester (SADBE), and diphencyprone (DCP); and (3) steroids.[77] Minoxidil, marketed as Rogaine, is also used to treat androgenetic alopecia: male and female pattern baldness.[78]

Minoxidil

Topical minoxidil, such as the well-known brand Rogaine, is a clear, watery solution applied directly to the scalp. It is reported to be effective with the regrowth of hair in about thirty percent of the people who use it, especially when the treatment regimen is followed as prescribed. For optimal results, patients are advised to apply the solution twice each day without fail. Should the treatment be stopped for any reason, progression of hair loss will resume and will be evident after about three months. This means that, for lasting results, Rogaine is a life-long treatment.[79]

Now available in a five percent, extra-strength, nonprescription solution, Rogaine was first introduced as an application for men's use only. Rogaine for Women is now on the market and is the exact same solution as is sold for men. Dawber and Van Neste say that the "effectiveness of topical minoxidil [Rogaine] in women with androgenetic alopecia is equivalent to the results seen in males," with some studies showing a success rate as high as fifty-five percent.[80]

How does Rogaine work? When hair follicles are in a dormant cycle (and shrinking), the hair stops growing. Daily applications of Rogaine will increase blood flow to the scalp,[81] nourish the anemic follicles, and motivate them to grow hair again.[82] Rogaine can thicken the hair in the front and on the sides of the head, but it works best on the bald spot on the crown. The hair around the frontal hairline is usually the first to go, leaving no salvageable hair (or follicles) for Rogaine to work on. The hair on the crown takes years to fall out completely and, perhaps for that reason, responds well to a hair follicle stimulant.[83] The process of hair follicle shrinkage to the point of no growth at all takes years; the sooner one begins to reverse the process, the better. Success is more likely to come to young men who start using Rogaine the moment they notice a thinning hairline or a tiny bald spot in the crown.[84]

Sensitizing Agents

Dinitrochlorobenzene (DNCB), squaric acid dibutyl ester (SADBE), and diphencyprone (DPC) are potent chemicals that are reported to have successfully generated the regrowth of hair in some individuals diagnosed with alopecia areata. Known as "topical contact sensitization" or "topical immunotherapy," this treatment is be-lieved to suppress the mechanisms that cause hair loss. The success-ful use of such chemicals, however, appears to be limited. It has worked well for some individuals experiencing hair loss and not at all for others. Dawber and Van Neste say that success with contact sensitization has been greatest when used in patchy alopecia areata, and "least in alopecia totalis [total loss of scalp hair] and alopecia universalis [loss of all body hair]."[85]

The treatment is also risky, as the chemicals are dangerous to work with. They have been known to cause blistering, rash, intense itching, and oozing, all of which can result in secondary infection.[86] When choosing this type of treatment, all precautions must be taken to protect the patient and the individuals (i.e., pharmacist, nurse, physician) handling the chemicals.

Steroids

Topical steroids can be used successfully on patchy alopecia areata and also on more extensive cases of hair loss. They are gener-ally supplied in a cream base and are applied twice each day to the affected sites. The extent of one's hair loss does not seem to be a factor in the success of this treatment, but age and duration of symp-toms do matter. Children seem to respond quite well to topical ste-roids (regardless of duration of symptoms), whereas adults do not if evidence of hair loss has been around longer than a year.[87]

Possible negative side effects from the use of topical steroids are inflammation of the hair follicles, acne, and hypertrichosis (excess hair growth). Also, if the amount applied to the scalp is too great or the prescribed strength of the medication is too high, systemic absorption is possible (along with accompanying un-pleasant side effects.)[88]

ORAL MEDICATIONS

finasteride

Finasteride (currently marketed under the brand name Propecia) is a relatively harmless antiandrogen preparation prescribed for the treatment of hair loss. Originally sold as Proscar (an agent to treat enlarged prostates), Propecia works by decreasing the male hormone dihydrotestosterone, which is linked to baldness and prostate tissue growth. When the body's level of dihydrotestosterone is reduced (by taking Propecia), the hair follicles are no longer affected by the hormone and they begin to sprout hair again.[89] Propecia is prescribed for men only at this time.

Another strategy is to use Rogaine and Propecia simultaneously. One drug (Rogaine) stimulates hair growth topically, and the other (Propecia) systemically decreases the hormone level that causes baldness. Some men, however, are avoiding Propecia altogether because of a few reported negative side effects: birth defects, especially if the child is male, have been reported (although some experts feel that this has been exaggerated) and a small percentage of participants complained of erectile dysfunction. One other less known side effect of Propecia is that it can slightly lower one's PSA (Prostatic Specific Antigen) results in a prostate cancer screening test, possibly masking a potentially serious problem.[90]

Spironolactone

Generally prescribed as a diuretic and a means to reduce high blood pressure (an antihypertensive), spironolactone appears to encourage the regrowth of hair in women diagnosed with androgenic alopecia. Like Propecia, spironolactone interferes with the production (and effect) of androgens, allowing hair follicles to resume a more normal growth cycle. At this time, all studies examining hair regrowth (using spironolactone) have only been performed in women, meaning that there are no reports in the literature on how effective the drug would be for men.[91]

Reported negative side effects for women taking spironolactone are an irregular menstrual cycle, mood swings, nausea, fatigue, headache, birth defects (particularly in a male fetus), and breast tenderness.[92] Men taking spironolactone (for high blood pressure) have reported impotence, decreased interest in sex, and enlarged breasts.[93] The possible side effects that accompany this drug are discouraging. For those reasons alone, one might understand why spironolactone is avoided as a treatment for hair loss.

Oral Steroid Preparations

The use of oral steroid preparations for the treatment of hair loss has shown some success, but the accompanying side effects are so unpleasant that it may not be worth the effort. Weight gain (in some cases, obesity) was the most frequently reported side effect, with other patients complaining of mood changes, acne, headaches, and menstrual difficulties.[94] In some cases, an individual taking oral steroids to combat hair loss may be trading one problem for another, especially if weight gain is the experienced side effect.

Drugs and Potions on the Horizon

Reports indicate that there are a large number of oral preparations (hormone inhibitors) and topical applications (follical stimulants) currently being tested in the laboratory, ones that are bearing the promise of hair regrowth. GlaxoSmithKline is reportedly having good success with an oral preparation in clinical trials, one that works similarly to Propecia.[95]

THE FUTURE OF GENE THERAPY IN THE TREATMENT OF HAIR LOSS

It's been known for some time that androgenetic alopecia runs in families. Rumor has it that the gene is passed through the mother to her son(s), or daughter(s) as the case may be, and a rumor is all that it's been. "Folklore . . ." says John Sedgewick. "Mothers are not solely responsible; fathers can pass along the trait, too."[96] However, little has been said about genetics and the search for a cure for the *follicly challenged*. That is, until now.

Angela Christiano — a genetic dermatologist who copes with hair loss herself — claims to have discovered the hairless gene, the one that causes an inherited form of alopecia. This discovery will hopefully open the door to a related treatment in the future.[97] Christiano's hope is to create a kind of genetic ointment that, when applied, will stimulate the dormant follicles.[98] Another researcher in the field has achieved some success with injecting genes into laboratory mice; the report is that the injections successfully produced active hair follicles — along with a nasty side effect of benign tumors.[99] It is, however, a beginning. Other genetic studies are surely in the making.

Hair loss has been a focus of social, psychological, and medical concern for thousands of years. Potions, pomades, and remedies to treat the condition during earlier times were brewed, stewed, and prayed over. As time passed, causes of baldness were suspected and identified, preventive measures were implemented and encouraged, and newer, more bearable treatments were recommended. Today, individuals have several choices when searching for ways to regrow hair. In more recent times, surgical procedures, oral preparations, injections, and potent follicle stimulators have come to the forefront.

Regardless of the cost, eventual outcome, postoperative pain, and possible complications, individuals who are balding will frequently choose surgical procedures in hopes of attaining more hair Often people who are losing their hair will go into debt, undergo the knife, endure long and uncomfortable convalescence . . . they will do just about anything to get their hair back.

Less radical treatments involve steroid injections, topical applications, and/or oral preparations. And there is promise for newer, more effective treatments. In teaching universities, pharmaceutical laboratories — perhaps even in someone's basement — research is ongoing, looking for a cure for baldness.

Clearly, hair is something to be proud of. Baldness remains a major concern for many.

CHAPTER TEN

HAIR PEACE

Wigs, Wigbands, Hair Extensions, Toupees,
Rugs, and Other Choices for
Finding a Little Hair Peace

SHEILA

Sheila entered my office with the confidence of a Miss America — and she was attractive, personable, and engaging enough to compete for that title. Having lost all of her hair at the age of three to alopecia universalis, Sheila schooled herself in applying make-up (including lashes and brows) and in choosing and wearing a wig.

> From the moment he became bald, Louis XIV never permitted himself to be seen without his wig by anyone save only Binette, his personal barber. Night and morning the King's wig had to be passed through the drawn curtains of his four-poster bed.
>
> — Pearl Binder

She pulls it off with grace and ease, this woman who saved herself from a society obsessed with physical attractiveness. She said it hadn't been easy:

Growing up I just got sick and tired of having to try on wigs, and do this and get that. But as I got older I said to myself, "this is just something I know I have got to have. This is part of me. I am going to have to do this every day until I die." Now they've improved hair pieces and I'm having a human hair wig made. It's being made just for me, and I think that adds to my confidence. So it's getting easier.[1]

Should she ever appear in public bareheaded, Sheila knows it would create a stir. "Look at that girl. Why is she doing that?" [mimicking others]. "I'd feel all right about it," she said, "but other people are going to make you feel uncomfortable."

> I work with a woman at the bank who had cancer, and she went through chemo and lost her hair, and she didn't wear a wig — and about this time she came back to work. It didn't bother her, but I noticed the way people would react to her. They didn't want to get too close, or they didn't want to talk with her like they had normally been doing. But when her hair started growing back, people started going out of their way to speak to her. They would hug her and smile. They kind of eased up. They would see her coming and meet her before she could get to them.[2]

The observation that differences can create uneasiness and distance among people began during Sheila's teenage years when she "felt like an outcast."[3] Her choice to don a wig and create eyebrows and lashes became an opportunity to feel better about herself, to feel more comfortable in society, and to be more attractive. The color of her hair, the length of her lashes, the shape of her brows are all within her control — a control she uses effectively to enhance her beauty and charm.

Women particularly feel self-conscious (even traumatized) when they lose their hair, and many look for some kind of hair replacement. Debbie, a cancer patient who lost her thick, blond hair as a result of radiation treatment, was especially affected by her baldness: she was in the beauty business — she sold cosmetics. Looking attractive was important in her line of work. At first she resisted buying a wig. She was at home during the early stages of recovery and had hoped that her hair would grow back during her confinement.

It didn't, and she gave in. She bought a wig — and for the first time in a long time, she looked forward to going out of the house. "Guys started looking at me again," she said. Having hair helped her look like her old self, and that made her feel normal.[4]

The *Perruque*

The term wig is from the French word *perruque*, which evolved over time into the words *perewig*, *perwig*, and finally *wig* (probably an English mispronunciation). Wigs have been important throughout history, but the English and fashionable French took it a step further. They developed an entire language around the wear and care of hair and the *perruque*. At one time, French gentlemen sat baldheaded in salons, while hairdressers curled their large and extravagant wigs with *bilboquets* (hot clay pipes). The men wore large hair, and the French women wore lovelocks — each ringlet bearing a flowerly name. Small curls over the forehead were *favourites*, side curls *confidantes*, and *creve-coeurs* described the ringlets over the ears.[5]

Wigs have been around for centuries; evidence of their use in ancient Egypt has turned up through the excavation of mummies and burial sites. Cooper said that "wigs of fabulous cost were interred with the wealthy dead, to act as symbols of affluence and importance even beyond the grave." She said that a "wig discovered with a mummy from the 26th dynasty (about 600 B.C.) was made of pure silver." Wigs were used as symbols of wealth and as disguises; in some parts of the world they were — and still are — used as emblems of different professions. Wigs have a long and colorful history in the theater and film industry,[6] and a stylish wig may forever accessorize a woman's fashionable wardrobe.

Advances in technology — especially the development of synthetic wigs — have made the acquisition of a new head of hair both desirable and affordable. In some cases, they have made such a purchase irresistible, especially for those individuals who are losing . . . hair. The full wig, wigbands, hair extensions, toupees, rugs, and other televised options — all offer ways to disguise baldness effectively.

The Full Wig

A full wig covers at least 80-90 percent of the hair-bearing scalp. Anything less is considered a toupee or rug (for men), or a wiglet, weave-in, or fall (for women). All wigs are categorized by what they are made of: animal hair,[7] human hair, synthetic hair — and the way the wig is tied (i.e., hand-tied or machine-tied) to the mesh cap.[8]

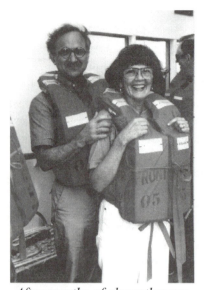

After months of chemotherapy, the author's dear friend, Rita Hillenbrand, on a cruise with her husband; she is wearing a new, hand-sewn, real-human-hair wig.

Animal hair is generally selected for silver and white wigs, whereas the hair of horses, monkeys, dogs, goats, or yaks is most often used for other colors.[9]

Wigs made of human hair are superior both in handling and in appearance, if the hair has never been permed, bleached, or colored in any way. A human hair wig is also more expensive.[10] The most expensive (and nicest) human-hair wigs are made of European hair — mainly because this type of hair is the easiest to manage. The less expensive human-hair wigs are made with Indonesian,[11] Indian, or Oriental hair — which tends to be coarse, more difficult to manage, and has a tendency to curl. Another consideration when shopping for a wig, says Jonathan Zizmore, is to not be fooled by where the wig was made:

The location of the wig factory does not mean that's where the hair came from. It is not uncommon for a wig advertised as "imported from France" to be made of inexpensive human hair from South Korea. And, by the same token, some excellent-quality European-hair wigs are, for reasons of cost, manufactured outside Europe.[12]

Hence, it is important to question the clerk (or owner of the salon) as to the type of hair used to make the wig, rather than trust the location of the factory.

Synthetic wigs are less expensive (generally under $100),[13] but they don't look as nice and do not hold up as well as a human-hair wig. Artificial hair tends to oxidize (how it reacts when it binds with oxygen), making the colors of a synthetic wig dull. (Human hair can react in the same way, but never to the degree that synthetic hair does.) Initially it's difficult to tell a human-hair wig from a brand-new synthetic one. Zizmore says that a sure test is to "pluck a single strand and hold it over a lighted match. A synthetic fiber will melt and form a bead; a strand of human hair will quickly frazzle and leave an unpleasant sulfurous odor."[14] It isn't reasonable, of course, to perform this test while shopping, but it is helpful to know if you've gotten what you paid for.

Wigs are also classified by how they are tied (attached to the net cap): by hand or by machine. Hand-tied wigs are advertised as easier to manage, and they are more expensive.[15] They look authentic because the hairs are tied to the cap individually (much like the way the hair grows), but this also makes the wig more delicate. Machine-tied wigs are usually more sturdy[16] and are believed to be as manageable as hand-tied wigs. They are also cheaper,[17] but they don't have the natural, loose appearance of a hand-tied wig.[18]

A human-hair wig is a serious investment, many costing well over $1,000. A human hair wig also needs professional maintenance (i.e., it should be washed, set, and styled in a beauty salon), generally after eight or ten wearings. If this type of wig is preferable, one really needs two wigs: a spare to wear while the other is being groomed. Air pollution and oils from the scalp are the two major culprits that contribute to the frequent need for upkeep of a human-hair wig. The less expensive synthetic wig can be maintained at home with regular shampoos.[19]

A wig will last according to the quality of the purchase and wear and tear. Most wigs last no longer than three years. When not in use, the well-cared-for wig is placed on a block — usually made of plastic and shaped like a human head. The well-cared-for wig is also protected from sunlight and dust; most are covered with something soft and light, like a thin scarf.[20]

The Wigband

The *wigband* — hair sewn onto a band of fabric — was popular in the 1960s. Synthetic or human air is first sewn onto a net (or mesh) cap, then finished around the edges with a stretchy, snug-fitting band.

Several advantages accompany this type of hair piece: (1) the *band* cleverly disguises the front edge of the wig; (2) it is relatively inexpensive; (3) for complete baldness, one can purchase a wigband with bangs; (4) it is simple to put on and arrange; and (5) it is comfortable and practical. Despite the 1960s popularity of the wigband, it may be difficult to find one today.[21]

Hair Extensions

The basic methods of extending hair (using a hair piece to add fullness and length to one's existing hair) are *weaving, bonding, infusion,* and *clip-ons* — with all methods requiring professional assistance (a beautician). According to Gale Hansen, the best hair dresser for you depends on the style you want and the condition of your hair.[22]

Hair weaving is accomplished by sewing pieces of synthetic or human hair onto the client's real hair. (Weaving is the method that Hattie selected when she noticed patches of baldness on her scalp. If you recall, in the early stages she tried pulling strands of hair over the bald spots and securing them with bobby pins, but the bald spots grew larger, and eventually she decided to hide them with a weave-in.[23])

With this procedure, the existing hair is parted into sections, then flat-braided (like cornrows). Next, color and type of hair is matched to the client's own hair. The strands or wefts of hair (longer than the client's own hair) are then carefully braided or sewn onto the real hair, as close to the scalp as possible. Cutting and styling follow, with the entire process taking from two to four hours. The cost of weaving varies considerably, ranging anywhere from $500 to $2,500.[24]

Several problems accompany the method of hair weaving. As the client's real hair grows, the weave-in loosens (moving away from the scalp with the growing hair), requiring an adjustment from time to time. A second problem involves cleanliness, as hair weaves can't be washed as often or as forcefully as a normal head of hair. A desired change in style also presents a problem, because it's impossible to make a change without undoing the weave.[25] Otherwise a weave-in is a good choice for those who are experiencing patches of baldness, like Hattie.

In *bonding*, wefts or pieces of hair are glued to the scalp or to wax that has been applied to the hair. It's a short-term style, lasting about one week. One drawback with bonding is that glue can damage the hair, even pull it out if extensions are removed carelessly. (The glue should be loosened and removed with baby oil before washing.) Bonding is a fairly inexpensive method (ranging from $50 to $250), and if done well, it can be a lifesaver for a fun, quick hairstyle for a special event,[26] especially if one's hair is thinning.

The *infusion, interlocking,* or *strand-by-strand* method of hair extension involves the wax-gluing of individual strands of hair to the client's own hair. It is accomplished with the aid of a special wax-glue gun and can last up to four months. Infusing takes time and can be as highly priced as weaving — but the result is a smoother, more natural look, a favorite method of many stylists. Some complain that the technique of infusion can cause hair to become brittle (and break), but others disagree, saying that there is less hair-pulling than with weaving or braiding. (Infusing can be accomplished more quickly by attaching small sections of preglued strands to the existing hair.)[27]

A *clip-on* is a thrust of hair that can be attached to one's existing hair with the use of pins, combs or clips. It lasts for a day or special evening.[28] Boasting a longer history than weaving, bonding, and infusion — clip-ons have been available for years, the most popular being a *wiglet* and a *fall*.

Clip-on hair pieces for women were originally called *toupees for women*, and were used in the early 1900s to help create the Gibson girl pompadour (a full and raised hair style of that era). During that time, hair accessories were being presented in a variety of fashions (i.e., switch, soft curled bangs, chignon, bun, braid)[29] and did much to achieve smart and fashionable hairdressing. During the mid to late 1960s the wiglet was introduced and was used to create a fuller hairstyle. The wiglet is simply a thrust of hair, usually short, attached to a circle of netting (4 to 5 inches in diameter) and held in place with bobby pins, clips, or combs, effectively adding thickness to a thinning head of hair. The wiglet can be a welcome asset for a woman who is experiencing diffuse hair loss.

A *fall* is a long, glamorous thrust of hair anchored to the existing hair (on the crown) with clips, pins, or small combs — creating the illusion of having long, thick, nicely styled tresses.[30] The mini-fall, the cascade, and the mini-mini-fall are simply shorter versions of this type of hairpiece, usually no longer than eight inches in length.[31] A fall is a good choice for someone whose hair is growing back in but hasn't yet reached a desirable length.

THE TOUPEE

During the eighteenth century, the word *foretop* was used to describe the hair, real or fake, just above the forehead. It was a style that was built up or raised — sometimes shooting straight up — and then descended slowly as it reached the crown. As this hairstyle (for men) grew in importance the foretop became known as the toupee;[32] over time the word toupee was used to describe a man's hairpiece — a hairpiece that became the makings of big business. According to Richard Corson, in the late 1950s one mail-order company sent out 30,000 catalogs in carefully disguised white envelopes "advertising their 'career-winning toupees'." They ranged in price from $109.95 to $224.95. Other companies followed suit, with one company boasting a "750 per cent increase in the sale of men's hairpieces." This flurry of activity around the toupee was, no doubt, bolstered by the knowledge that many male movie stars (and television actors) were known to wear them.[33]

A toupee resembles a wiglet but is usually held in place with special tape or glue — not an effective means of securing a hairpiece, as there's always the fear that perspiration will loosen the adhesive, causing one's hair to shift out of place, or even take flight on a windy day. Toupees are still available, but they are not as practical a choice for men as newer options for a hairpiece purchase.

During the early 1970s the *rug* was introduced, offering balding males a more natural looking (and more secure) head of hair. (A rug is the male version of a weave-in.) With this technique, a portion of the client's existing hair is braided, providing a woven base to which hair pieces are attached with nylon thread (lending greater reinforcement than glue or tape). Men who choose this method of hair replacement can swim or shower, even participate in sports without the fear of exposing a bald head. Yet there are problems — similar to those experienced by women who have a weave-in: As the braided hair grows, the hair piece will shift away from the scalp, requiring an adjustment every two to three months; initial and maintainance costs are excessive; aggravated dandruff conditions are likely; and further hair loss has been reported.

In the 1980s, new and improved ways of replacing hair came to the forefront — innovative ways that presented fewer unwanted side effects, and reported by users to be highly successful.[34]

Televised Options

We have all seen advertisements on TV — those carefully crafted ads convincing balding males that, not only can they can have a new head of glorious hair they can have everything that comes with it: beautiful women, athletic ability, and instant popularity. (The models they use are young, muscular, happy, and downright handsome.) Regardless of the subtle ploy for secondary gain, some of these brilliantly marketed ways of hiding baldness do offer an instant head of hair.

First, the services are explained — services that involve matching, weaving, gluing, styling, restyling and replacement.

Next, human hair is matched to the client's own hair in color and texture. These longer strands of hair are then woven onto a plastic, web-like structure. The top of the head is shaved, and the rim of the cap is glued onto the scalp. A trim and style follow, one that matches the client's favorite hairstyle (copied from an earlier snapshot).[35]

One generally pays between $1,600 to $2,700 for such a procedure. This covers the hairpiece (also called a rug), initial styling, and a 90-day guarantee (approximately). The cost is paid up front, and only half is refundable should the client be dissatisfied. A maintenance program is offered (approximately $199/month as a monthly fee) because the hairpiece usually requires regular styling, and must be replaced periodically (usually every three months).[36]

What Lies Beneath

Wearing a wig or hairpiece doesn't suit everyone. Some individuals, like Yolanda, say that a wig is uncomfortable. She said it was so tight it gave her a headache. A wig can also be hot, depending on the fabric of the mesh cap (and season of the year). A net cap made from a lighter fabric (i.e., silk) is cooler, but a heavier fabric (i.e., cotton) will hold its shape longer.[37] And, as mentioned, a wig can be too tight. (Yet, if it isn't tight enough, it can slide around too easily.) Another reported reason for refusing to wear a wig or hairpiece is that — emotionally and psychologically — it simply may not feel right.

Wearing a wig didn't work for Amy Spindler — a style editor with the *New York Times Magazine* — and for reasons other than comfort. A cancer survivor who lost her hair during chemotherapy, Amy quickly purchased a wig that was identical to her own hair. But when she tried it on, she cried: "Not because it wasn't totally real; it was. But I didn't feel like that dark-haired, dour person with the shaggy hair anymore." Amy sent the wig back to have highlights sewn in, but the result was still dissatisfying: "Putting on that cloak of hair was a reminder of everything I'd been doing in my lifestyle that I felt had given me cancer."[38]

> Something strange had happened to me, psychologically, on my way to becoming cancer-free. I'd reclaimed my life, how screwed up my priorities were, how hard I was working. It wasn't only my entire closet full of Ann Demeulemeester black suits that didn't seem to fit who I was anymore: my hair didn't either.[39]

Amy purchased several wigs but only wore them occasionally. She preferred hats and at times got in touch with her "inner punk": no hair, a magnetic stud that she wore on her lip (or nose), weird earrings, and a lot of makeup. Amy completed her radiation treatments, and one week later married her devoted fiance. She reports that her hair has grown back in.[40]

Renata Polt, another cancer survivor, purchased three wigs before her hair fell out (a recommendation of the American Cancer Society), each a different style and color. Her husband assured her that she looked attractive in them, but Renata only wore them a few times. Instead she wore scarves, caps, and berets (mostly for warmth), and at times she simply let her scalp "hang out." A vacation in Hawaii prompted Renata to go public with her bare head:

> We had no sooner landed in Honolulu than I removed my

cap and stuffed it into my bag. I don't remember a more liberating moment in my life. I stood up straighter, held my head higher, and felt as if I'd been let out of a cage. And nobody stared. Once or twice during our nine days' stay, strangers — women, invariably — would come up to me and say, 'Have you had chemo? I had it a couple of years ago, and now I'm fine, and you will be too.' Along with my sense of liberation came a resurgence of energy, and when I got back home I felt like, well, like myself again.[41]

Renata was glad to be alive, happy to be inside a healing and intact body. She began to love and respect every part of herself in ways that she never imagined possible. "My head was going to be part of me," she said, "hair or no hair." Renata's hair would grow back in, of course. But during her experience of hair loss, she respected it as part of the healing process, she honored her self (her feelings, needs, and desires), and she valued her life above all.[42]

Men, too, vary on the scale of desiring a hairpiece. Not all balding men react negatively to losing their hair,[43] so it stands to reason that these individuals would not attempt to cover it up. Dave wasn't particularly bothered by his hair loss, and he did not seem interested in replacing it. During our meeting he had not ruled out a transplant or a hairpiece, but neither of those choices was "on the front burner." He didn't enjoy the idea of looking older, but other than that he seemed perfectly comfortable with his hair loss.[44]

༄

The wearing of wigs can be traced back to the ancient Egyptians where they once served as symbols for the elite (the greater the wealth, the fancier the wig). The nicest wigs were made of human hair, although some were made of lavish material and sometimes trimmed with beads. Such wigs signified power and affluence and were buried with their owners as symbols of such. Hence, it is from ancient Egyptian burial sites as well as paintings and sculpture, that we learn of the importance of wigs during earlier times.

Because hair loss can be a painful emotional problem, it isn't surprising that many individuals — both men and women — opt for a wig or hairpiece to remedy the situation. Wigs, hair extensions, toupees, and rugs are available and affordable. Women often purchase a wig or hair extension not to cover hair loss but simply to accessorize their wardrobe.

Shopping for a wig or hairpiece can be fun. It can be an enjoyable, entertaining, and worthwhile adventure, if the search is simply to accessorize the wardrobe. If one is shopping to cover hair loss that is the result of a serious illness or aggressive treatment . . . it's an entirely different matter.

I send my warmest wishes to all of you.

NOTES

Introduction

1   Judi Johnson and Linda Klein, *I Can Cope, Staying Healthy With Cancer* (Minneapolis, MN: Chronimed Publishing, 1994), p. 123; Selma Schimmel with Barry Fox, *Cancer Talk* (New York, NY: Broadway Books, 1999), p. 58.

2   B. G. Campbell, *Human Evolution, An Introduction to Man's Adaptations* (Chicago: Aldine Publishing Company, 1966); Charles Darwin, *The Origin of the Species and the Descent of Man* (New York: The Modern Library, 1936); C. B. Goodhart, "The Evolutionary Significance of Human Hair Patterns and Skin Coloring," *Advancement of Science* (1960), 17:53–59.

3   Desmond Morris, *The Naked Ape* (London: Jonathan Cape, 1967), p. 43; Campbell, *Human Evolution*, p. 238.

4   W. Montagna, "The Skin," *Scientific America* (1965) 212:53–59.

5   E. Hatfield and S. Sprecher, *Mirror, Mirror . . . the Importance of Looks in Everyday Life* (Albany: State University of New York Press, 1986).

6   C. Willette Cunnington, *Feminine Attitudes in the Nineteenth Century* (New York: Haskell House Publishers Ltd., 1973); James Laver, *Taste and Fashion* (London: George G. Harrap and Company Ltd, 1945); Timothy Miller, *The Hippies and American Values* (Knoxville: The University of Tennessee Press, l991); Charlotte Yonge, *Womankind* (New York: Macmillan and Company, 1882).

7   T. Ryback, "Evidence of Evil," *The New Yorker*, November 15, 1993, pp. 68–81.

8   J. Andresen, "Rapunzel: The Symbolism of the Cutting of Hair," *The Journal of the American Psychoanalytic Association* (1980) 28(1):68-88; C. Berg, "The Unconscious Significance of Hair," The International Journal of Psychoanalysis (1951) 17:73–88; P. Hershman, "Hair, Sex and Dirt," Man, (N.S.) (1974) 9:275–298.

9   P. Gundry, *Woman Be Free* (Grand Rapids, MI: Zondervan Publishing House, 1988).

10   R. Firth, *Symbols, Public and Private* (Ithaca, NY: Cornell University Press, 1973).

11   Wendy Cooper, *Hair, Sex, Society, Symbolism* (New York: Stein and Day, 1971), p. 196.

12   Ibid., p. 24.

Chapter One — The Spread of the Peacock's Tail

1   C. Darwin, *The Origin of the Species and the Descent of Man* (New York: The Modern Library, 1936), p. 431.
2   W. Cooper, *Hair, Sex, Society, Symbolism* (New York: Stein and Day, 1971).
3   W. Montagna, "The Skin," *Scientific America* (1965) 212:53–59.
4   Cooper, *Hair*, p. 13.
5   Bernard Campbell, *Human Evolution: An Introduction to Man's Adaptations* (Chicago: Aldine Publishing Company, 1966), p. 238; Cooper, *Hair*, p. 16.
6   D. Morris, *The Naked Ape* (New York: McGraw-Hill, 1967), p. 43; Campbell, *Human Evolution*, p. 238.
7   Darwin, *Origin of the Species*; C. B. Goodhart, "The Evolutionary Significance of Human Hair Patterns and Skin Coloring," *Advancement of Science* (1960) 17:53-59; Montagna, "The Skin," pp. 53–59; Morris, *The Naked Ape*.
8   Darwin, *Origin of the Species*, p. 69.
9   Ibid.
10 Helen Fisher, *Anatomy of Love* (New York: W.W. Norton and Company, 1992), p.181.
11 Goodhart, "The Evolutionary Significance," p. 53.
12 Campbell, *Human Evolution*, p. 239.
13 Goodhart, "The Evolutionary Significance," p. 53.
14 Ibid
15 Ibid., p. 54.
16 Cooper, *Hair*, p. 65.
17 Campbell, *Human Evolution*, p. 264.
18 Cooper, *Hair*, p. 65.
19 Fisher, *Anatomy of Love*, p. 20.
20 Darwin, *Origin of Species*, p. 907.
21 Goodhart, "The Evolutionary Significance," p. 54.
22 Fisher, *Anatomy of Love*, p. 180.
23 Charles Darwin, *The Descent of Man and Selection in Relation to Sex* (New York: Modern Library, 1871), p. 907.

Chapter Two — Wavelengths

1   Sara Romweber, *Understanding the Emotional Experience of Scalp Hair Loss*. Ph.D. doctoral dissertation, Saybrook Institute, San Francisco, CA, 1996.
2   C. Willett Cunnington, *Feminine Attitudes in the Nineteenth Century* (New York: Haskell House Publishers Ltd., 1973), p.166.
3   J. Laver, *Taste and Fashion* (London: George G. Harrap and Company LTD, 1945), p. 115.
4   Richard Corson, *Fashions in Hair* (London: Peter Owen Limited, 1965), pp. 497–559.
5   Cunnington, *Feminine Attitudes*, pp. 166–168.
6   Charlotte Yonge, *Womankind* (New York: Macmillan and Co., 1882), p. 112.
7   Ibid.

8   Paul Poiret, "Individuality in Dress, The Secret of the Well-Dressed Woman," in *Harper's Bazaar*, ed. Jane Trahey (New York: Random House, 1967), p. 12.
9   Corson, *Fashions in Hair*, p. 608 and p. 613.
10 Cooper, *Hair*, pp. 76–77.
11 Corson, *Fashions in Hair*, p. 613.
12 Laver, *Taste and Fashion*, p. 125.
13 Corson, *Fashions in Hair*, p. 600.
14 Laver, *Taste and Fashion*, pp. 212–221.
15 Maria Aldrich, "Hair," in *The Best American Essays 1993*, ed. Joseph Epstein (New York: Ticknor and Fields, l993), pp. 2–3.
16 Cooper, *Hair*, p. 135.
17 Diane Ackerman, *A Natural History of Love* (New York: Random House, 1994), p. 190.
18 R. Firth, *Symbols, Public and Private* (Ithaca, NY: Cornell University Press, 1973), p. 274.
19 Ackerman, *Natural History of Love*, p. 192.
20 Aldrich, "Hair," pp. 3–4.
21 L. Caligor and R. May, *Dreams and Symbols, Man's Unconscious Language* (New York: Basic Books, Inc., 1968), p. 105.
22 Aldrich, "Hair," p. 1.
23 Janice Min, Joel Stratte-McClure, Cathy Nolan, Nina Biddle, and Toula Vlahou, "Trouble in Monaco," *People* (September 30, 1996), pp. 71–76.
24 Corson, *Fashions in Hair*, p. 398.
25 Ibid., p. 404.
26 Ibid., pp. 405–408.
27 Alexander Rowland, *The Human Hair* (London, 1853), quoted in Corson, *Fashions in Hair*, p. 407.
28 Unknown source from Irish Quarterly, quoted in Corson, *Fashions in Hair*, p. 408.
29 Cooper, *Hair*, p. 43.
30 Laver, *Taste and Fashion*, p. 188.
31 Cunnington, *Feminine Attitudes*, p. 4.
32 Corson, *Fashions in Hair*, p. 420.
33 Ibid., p. 560.
34 Firth, *Symbols*, p. 277.
35 Corson, *Fashions in Hair*, p. 577.
36 Ibid., pp. 580–581.
37 Ibid., p. 582.
38 Firth, *Symbols*, p. 276.
39 Ibid., p. 277.
40 Miller, *The Hippies and American Values*, p. 116.
41 A. Synnott, "Shame and Glory: A Sociology of Hair . . ." *British Journal of Sociology* (1987)38(3):381–413.
42 Miller, *Hippies and American Values*, pp. 116–117.
43 Firth, *Symbols*, p. 271.
44 Henry Finck, *Romantic Love and Personal Beauty* (New York: The Macmillan Company, 1912), p. 494.

45 Romweber, *Understanding the Emotional Experience*, pp. 114–146.

46 Tom Cash, "Losing Hair, Losing Points? The Effects of Male Pattern Baldness on Social Impression Formation . . ." *Journal of Applied Social Psychology* (1990) 20:154–167.

47 Michael Wogalter and Judith Hosie, "Effects of Cranial and Facial Hair on Perceptions of Age and Person . . ." *The Journal of Social Psychology* (1991) 131(4):589–591.

48 Allan Fenigstein, "Self-Consciousness, Self-Attention, and Social Interaction . . ." *Journal of Personality and Social Psychology* (1979) 37:75–86; Michael Sheier, "Effects of Public and Private Self-Consciousness on the Public Expression of Personal Beliefs . . ." *Journal of Personality and Social Psychology* (1980) 39(3):514–521.

49 Romweber, *Understanding the Emotional Experience*, pp. 114–143.

50 W. Walster, V. Aronson, D. Abrahams, and L. Rottman, "Importance of physical attractiveness in dating behavior . . ." *Journal of Personality and Social Psychology* (1966) 4:308–316; R. Brislin and S. Lewis, "Dating and Physical Attractiveness: Replication . . ." *Psychological Reports* (1968) 22:976.

Chapter Three — Rapunzel, Rapunzel . . .

1 Robert D. Nye. *Three Psychologies: Perspectives from Freud, Skinner, and Rogers.* (Monterey, CA: Brooks/Cole Publishing Company, 1981).

2 P. Zimbardo and F. Ruch. *Psychology and Life* (Glenview, IL: Scott Foresman and Company, 1977).

3 Berg, "The Unconscious Significance of Hair," pp. 73–88.

4 Ibid.

5 J. Grimm and W. Grimm, "Rapunzel," in *The Complete Grimm's Fairy Tales* (New York: Pantheon Books, 1944).

6 Andresen, "Rapunzel: The Symbolism of the Cutting of Hair," pp. 68–88.

7 Ibid.

8 M. D. Eder, "A Note on Shingling," *International Journal of Psychoanalysis* (1925) 6:325–326.

9 E. R. Leach, "Magical Hair," *Journal of the Royal Anthropological Institute* (1957) 88 (Part 2): 147–164.

10 Ibid., p. 149.

11 M. Douglas, *Natural Symbols* (London: The Cresset Press, 1970).

12 Leach, "Magical Hair," p. 151.

13 Ibid., pp. 154–155.

14 P. Hershman. "Hair, Sex, and Dirt," *Man* (N.S.) (1974) 9:275–298.

15 Ibid., p. 274.

16 Ibid., p. 275.

17 Ibid.

18 Ibid., pp. 277–278.

19 Ibid., p. 282.

20 Ibid., pp. 280–281.

21 Ibid., p. 280.

22 Margaret Williamson, "Powhatan Hair," *Man* (1979) 49(3):392–419.
23 Ibid., p. 398.
24 Ibid., pp. 405–406.
25 Ibid., p. 403.
26 Ibid., p. 406.
27 Ibid., p. 408.
28 Ibid., p. 395.
29 Esi Sagay, *African Hairstyles* (Portsmouth, New Hampshire: Heinemann, 1983).
30 Ibid., p. 20.
31 Ibid., p. 42.
32 Ibid., p.6.
33 Williamson, "Powhatan Hair," p. 395.
34 Leach, "Magical Hair," p. 160.

Chapter Four — Crown and Glory

1 Penny Chapman and Sue Masters (Executive Producers), and Ken Cameron (Director), *Brides of Christ* [Film] (Santa Sabina College, Sydney, New Southy Wales, Australia: Australian Broadcasting Corporation and Roadshow Coate and Carroll, 1991).
2 Patricia Gundry, *Woman Be Free* (Grand Rapids, Michigan: Zondervan Publishing House, 1977).
3 W. Crooke, *Folklore of Northern India* (Nai Sarak, Delhi: Munshiram Manoharlal, 1896), p. 66.
4 Christopher A. Faraone, *Talisman and Trojan Horses* (Oxford University Press: New York, 1992), p. 80; George Lyman Kittredge, *Witchcraft in Old New England* (Cambridge, MA: Harvard University Press, 1929), p. 90; Walter W. Skeat, *Malay Magic* (London: Frank Cass & Co. LTD., 1965), pp. 44–45.
5 Susan Schneider, *Jewish and Female* (New York: Simon and Schuster, 1984), pp. 234–240.
6 L. Scanzoni and N. Hardesty, *All We're Meant To Be* (Nashville, TN: Abingdon Press, 1986), p. 82.
7 Schneider, *Jewish and Female*, pp. 234–240.
8 Leo Trepp, *The Complete Book of Jewish Observance* (New York: Behrman House, Inc./Summit Books, 1980), p. 281.
9 Ibid.
10 Schneider, *Jewish and Female*, pp. 234–240.
11 Ibid., p. 240.
12 Ibid., p. 238.
13 Ibid., p. 239.
14 Genesis (24:65) in *The Torah, The First Five Books of Moses* (Philadelphia: The Jewish Publication Society of America, 1962), p. 42.
15 Theodor H. Gastor, *The Holy and the Profane* (New York: William Sloane Associates Publishers, 1955), p. 103.
16 Schneider, *Jewish and Female*, p. 236.
17 Jan Goodwin, *Price of Honor, Muslim Women Lift the Veil of Silence on the*

Islamic World (Boston, MA: Little, Brown and Company, 1994), p. 79.

18   Martha Lee is young American woman who converted to Islam in 1985. She embraces Islamic traditions, including hair covering. She is the daughter of one of my close friends.

19   Geraldine Brooks, *Nine Parts of Desire: The Hidden World of Islamic Women* (New York: Doubleday, 1995), p. 20.

20   *The Qur'an* (Surah, XXXIII: 53), translated by M. H. Shakir (Elmhurst, New York: Tahrike Tarsile Qur'an, Inc., 1993), p. 281.

21   *The Koran* (24:30), translated by N. J. Dawood (New York: Penguin Books, 1974), p. 248.

22   Naila Minai, *Women in Islam, Tradition and Transition in the Middle East* (New York: Seaview Books, 1981), p. xii.

23   Goodwin, *Price of Honor*, p. 105.

24   Ibid., p. 107.

25   Goodwin, *Price of Honor*, p. 9.

26   Ibid., p. 30.

27   Ibid., p. 8.

28   Minai, *Women in Islam*, p. xii.

29   Brooks, *Nine Parts of Desire*, p. 24.

30   Ibid., p. 20.

31   Ibid., p. 9.

32   Ibid., p. 30.

33   Minai, *Women in Islam*, p. 116.

34   Ibid.

35   Goodwin, *Price of Honor*, p. 8.

36   Suzanne Campbell-Jones, *In Habit, An Anthropological Study of Working Nuns* (London: Faber & Faber, 1979), p. 175.

37   Manuela Dunn-Mascetti, *Saints, The Chosen Few* (New York: Ballantine Books, 1994).

38   Cooper, *Hair, Sex, Society, Symbolism* , p. 129.

39   Marcel Bernstein, *The Nuns* (Philadelphia: J. B. Lippincott, 1976), p. 92.

40   Campbell-Jones, *In Habit*, p. 174.

41   Bernstein, *The Nuns*, p. 34.

42   Mary Gilligan Wong, *Nun, A Memoir of Mary Gilligan Wong* (San Diego: Harcourt Brace Jovanovich Publishers, 1983), p. 203.

43   Ibid., p. 203.

44   Midge Turk, *The Buried Life* (New York: The World Publishing Company, 1971), p. 50.

45   Ibid., pp. 50–51.

46   Tsultrim Allione, *Women of Wisdom* (London: Routledge & Kegan Paul, 1984), p. 137.

47   "The First Epistle of Paul the Apostle to the Corinthians," *The Holy Bible, Revised Standard Version* (New York: Collins, 1973), p. 163.

48   C. Craig, "The First Epistle to the Corinthians," in *The Interpreter's Bible*, eds. G. Buttrick, W. Bowie, J. Knox, N. Harmon, P. Sherer, S. Terrien (New York: Abingdon-Cokesbury Press, 1953), p. 125.

49   "The First Epistle of Paul the Apostle to the Corinthians," *The Holy Bible*, p. 163.

50 Craig, *The Intepreters Bible*, pp.125–126.

51 Ibid., p. 127.

52 Gundry, *Woman Be Free*, p. 23.

53 J. Duncan M. Derrett, "Religious Hair," *Man* (N.S.), 1973, 8, pp. 100–103.

54 Paul Toews, *Mennonites in American Society*, 1930-1970 (Scottdale, Pennsylvania: Herald Press, 1996), p. 59.

55 Oscar Burkholder, quoted in Paul Toews, *Mennonites in American Society*, p. 59.

56 Cooper, *Hair*, p.188; Cullen Murphy, *The World According to Eve* (New York: Houghton Mifflin Company, 1998), pp. 110–111.

57 Cooper, *Hair*, pp. 186–187.

58 Gastor, *The Holy and the Profane*, p. 106.

59 E. R. Leach, "Magical Hair," *Journal of the Royal Anthropological Institute*, 1957, 88 (Part II):147-164.

60 Gastor, *The Holy and the Profane*, p. 106.

61 Cooper, *Hair*, p. 38.

62 a Malayo-Polynesian speaking people inhabiting the Celebes.

63 J. G. Frazier, *The Golden Bough, a Study in Magic and Religion*, vol. 2 (New York: McMillan & Co., 1940), p. 232.

64 Ibid., p. 233.

65 Frazier, *The Golden Bough*, p. 232.

66. E. Crawley, *The Mystic Rose*, vol. 1 (London: Boni and Liveright, 1927), p. 336.

67 Gastor, *The Holy and the Profane*, p. 107.

68 Ibid., pp. 66–67.

69 Ibid., p. 106.

70 Frazier, *The Golden Bough*, pp. 230–231

71 Richard Corson, *Fashions in Hair* (London: Peter Owen Limited, 1965), p. 28.

72 Ibid., p. 71.

73 Cooper, *Hair*, p. 183.

74 A. S. Gregor, *Witchcraft and Magic* (New York: Charles Scribner's Sons, 1972), pp. 9–12.

75 Kittredge, *Witchcraft*, p. 90.

76 Faraone, *Talisman and Trojan Horses*, p. 80.

77 Crawley, The Mystic Rose; *Frazier, The Golden Bough*; P. Bohannon, Edward B. Tylor: *Researches into the Early History of Mankind* (Chicago: The University of Chicago Press, 1938).

78 Corson, *Fashions in Hair*, p. 28.

79 Gregor, *Witchcraft and Magic*, p. 13.

80 Bohannon, *Edward B. Tylor*, p. 112.

81 Skeat, *Malay Magic*, pp. 44–45.

82 Cooper, *Hair*, p. 197.

83 Crooke, *Folklore of Northern India*, p. 281.

84 Moncure D. Conway, *Demonology and Devil-Lore* (London: Ballantyne Press, 1879), p. 91.

85 Ibid., p. 93.

86 Ibid., p. 96.
87 Ibid., p. 97.
88 Ibid., p. 98.
89 Gastor, *The Holy and the Profane*, p. 105.
90 James B. Hurley, *Man and Woman in Biblical Perspective* (Grand Rapids, Michigan: Zondervan Publishing House, 1981), p. 169.

Chapter Five — The Mane Attraction

1 S. Field and K. McCormick (Producers), and J. Schumacher (Director), *Dying Young* [Film]. (Hollywood, California: 20th Century Fox, 1991).
2 Ibid.
3 D. Ackerman, *A Natural History of Love* (New York: Random House, 1994), pp. 192–193.
4 Crooke, *Folklore of Northern India*, p. 67.
5 Ackerman, *A Natural History of Love*, p. 190.
6 John Lennon and Paul McCartney (Composers), "Here, There and Everywhere" [song] (Mayfair, London: Northern Songs Limited, 1966).
7 Lord Byron, "Maid of Athens, Ere We Part," *Romantic Poetry of the Early Nineteenth Century* (New York: Charles Scribner's Sons, 1928), p. 282.
8 Lord Byron, "She Walks in Beauty," *Romantic Poetry of the Early Nineteenth Century* (New York: Charles Scribner's Sons, 1928), p. 283.
9 Ackerman, *A Natural History of Love*, p. 190.
10 Cooper, *Hair: Sex, Society, Symbolism*, p. 38.
11 J. J. Lamorreaia, "Great Comebacks," in *Essence* (April, 1993), pp. 75–76.
12 R. Freedman, *Beauty Bound* (Lexington, MA: D. C. Heath and Company, 1986), pp. 28–29.
13 Dalma Heyn, "Are You Your Hair?" *Self*, February, 1997, p. 128.
14 N. Wolf, *The Beauty Myth* (New York: William Morrow and Company, 1991), p. 205.
15 Freedman, *Beauty Bound*, p. 74.
16 Heyn, "Are You Your Hair?" p. 129.
17 A. Corbin, *Le Miasme et la Jonquille* [The Foul and the Fragrant] (Paris: Aubier Montaigne, 1982), p. 43.
18 W. Montagna, "The Sebaceous Glands in Man," in *Advances in Biology of Skin*, eds. W. Montagna, R. Ellis, and A. Silver (New York: The Macmillan Company, 1963), pp. 19–31.
19 D. M. Stoddard, *The Scented Ape* (New York: Cambridge University Press, 1990), p. 52.
20 K. Wright, "The Sniff of Legend," *Discover* (April, 1994), p. 62.
21 Ibid., p. 64
22 Ibid.
23 Stoddard, *Scented Ape*, pp. 120–121.
24 Desmond Morris, *The Naked Ape* (London: Jonathan Cape, 1967), p. 76.
25 Ibid.
26 Ibid.

27   Havelock Ellis, *Psychology of Sex: A Manual for Students* (New York: Emerson Books, 1938), p. 97.

28   Al-Mutanabbi, "Verses composed in the poet's youth," in *Poems of Al-Mutanabbi*, translated by A. J. Arberry (Great Britain: Cambridge University Press, 1967), p. 18.

29   Cooper, *Hair*, p. 222.

30   Henry W. Boynton (Ed.), *The Complete Poetical Works of Pope* (New York: Houghton Mifflin Company, 1931), p. 91.

31   Ackerman, *A Natural History of Love*, p. 190.

Chapter Six — A Private and Silent Mourning

1   B. Simos, *A Time to Grieve* (New York: Family Service Association of America, 1979), p.11.

2   Ibid., pp. 11–12.

3   J. Barone, "Coping With Hair Loss," *Better Homes and Gardens*, September 1997, p. 105.

4   J. Lamorreaia, "Great Comebacks," *Essence*, April l993, p. 76.

5   Renata Polt, "Hair Apparent," *American Health*, June 1994, p. 18.

6   Ibid.

7   Romweber, *Understanding the Emotional Experience of Hair Loss.*

8   Simos, *A Time to Grieve*, p. 20; Barone, "Coping With Hair Loss," *Better Homes and Gardens*, September, 197, p. 105.

9   L. Festinger, "A Theory of Social Comparison Processes," *Human Relations* (1954) 7:117-140.

10   Neil Sadick and Donald Richardson, *Your Hair, Helping to Keep It* (Yonkers, New York: Consumer Reports Books, 1991), p. 3.

11   Ira Tanner, *The Gift of Grief* (New York: Hawthorne Books, Inc., 1976), p. 66.

12   Ibid., p. 116.

13   Ibid., p. 66.

14   Simos, *A Time to Grieve*, p. 62.

15   Ibid., pp. 52–53.

16   Suzanne M. Miller, "Why Having Control Reduces Stress: If I Can Stop the Roller Coaster, I Don't Want to Get Off," in *Human Helplessness, Theory and Applications*, eds. Judy Garber and Martin Seligman (New York: Academic Press, 1980), pp. 71–95.

17   Simos, *A Time to Grieve*, p. 161.

18   Ibid., pp. 160–161.

19   Tanner, *Gift of Grief*, p. 78.

20   Jack Miller, *The Healing Power of Grief* (New York: The Seabury Press, 1978), p. 58.

21   Ibid., p. 46.

22   Simos, *A Time to Grieve*, p. 127.

23   Richard Lazarus, *Psychological Stress and the Coping Process* (New York: McGraw-Hill Book Company, 1966), p. 265.

24   Barbara Sourkes, "A Life of My Own," in *The Deepening Shade: Psychologi-*

cal Aspects of Life Threatening Illness (Pittsburgh: University of Pittsburgh Press, 1982), p. 104

25   Sadick and Richardson, *Your Hair*, p. 1.

26   Cooper, *Hair, Sex, Society, Symbolism*, p. 74.

27   Simos, *A Time to Grieve*, p. 20.

28   Sadick and Richardson, *Your Hair*, p. 137.(description of weave-in).

29   Polt, "Hair Apparent," p. 22.

30   Miller, *The Healing Power of Grief*, p 10.

31   Polt, "Hair Apparent," p. 23.

32   Roxane Silver and Camille Wortman, "Coping with Undesirable Life Events," in *Human Helplessness, Theory and Applications*, eds. Judy Garber and Martin Seligman (New York: Academic Press, 1980), p.339.

33   Sadick and Richardson, *Your Hair*, p. 1–2.

34   R.W. Brislin, and S. A. Lewis, "Dating and physical attractiveness," *Psychological Reports*, 1968, 22:976; A. Tesser and M. Brodie, "A Note on Evaluation of a 'Computer Date,'" *Psychonomic Science* (1971) 23:300; E. Walster, V. Aronson, D. Abrahams, and L. Rottman, "The Importance of Physical Attractiveness in Dating Behavior," *Journal of Personality and Social Psychology* (1966) 4: 508–516.

35   Silver and Wortman, "Coping with Undesirable Life Events," p. 339.

36   Ibid.

37   Tanner, *The Gift of Grief*, pp.157–167.

38   Ibid., p. 115.

Chapter Seven — Survival Skills

1   Albert Ellis, *How to Control Your Anger Before it Controls You* (Sebaucus, NJ: Carol Publishing Group, 1997), p. 32.

2   Ibid., p. 31.

3   Robert A. Baron and Donn Byrne, *Social Psychology: Understanding Human Interaction* (Boston: Allyn and Bacon, 1981), p. 91.

4   Gerald Jampolsky and Diane Cirincione, *Change Your Mind, Change Your Life* (New York, NY: Bantam Books, 1993), pp. 18–19.

5   Baron and Byrne, *Social Psychology*, p. 134.

6   Marsha Linehan, *Skills Training Manual for Treating Borderline Personality Disorder* (New York: Guilford Press, 1993), p. 95.

7   Ibid.

8   Lamorreaia, "Great Comebacks," p, 76.

9   Maya Pines, "Psychological Hardiness: The Role of Challenge in Health," *Psychology Today* (December 1980), pp. 34–35.

10   Willie Jolley, *A Setback is a Setup for a Comeback* (New York: St. Martins Press, 1999), p. 19.

11   Pines, "Psychological Hardiness," pp. 34–35.

12   Norman Cousins, *Anatomy of an Illness as Perceived by the Patient* (New York: W.W. Norton, 1979), pp. 82–87.

13   Selma Schimmel and Barry Fox, *Cancer Talk: Voices of Hope and Endurance*

from "The Group Room," the World's Largest Cancer Support Group (New York: Broadway Books, 1999), p. 105.

14 Ibid., pp. 107–108.

15 Dave Beswick, *Bald Men Always Come Out on Top: 101 Ways to Use Your Head and Win with Skin* (St. Augustine, FL: Ama Publishing, 1997).

16 Jennifer Louden, *The Woman's Comfort Book* (San Francisco: Harper, 1992), p. 81.

17 Schimmel and Fox, *Cancer Talk*, p. 105.

18 Patricia Lynden interviewing Loretta LaRoche, "Queen of the Stress Busters," *New Age* (March/April 2001), p. 74.

19 Joseph Wolpe (with David Wolpe), *Our Useless Fears* (Boston: Houghton Mifflin, 1981), p. 8.

20 Sara Romweber, *Understanding the Emotional Experience of Hair Loss*, doctoral dissertation, Saybrook Graduate School and Research Center, San Francisco, CA, 1996.

21 Ibid.

22 Wolpe, *Our Usless Fears*, pp. 13–26.

23 Ibid., pp. 6–7.

24 Robert D. Nye, *Three Psychologies: Perspectives from Freud, Skinner, and Rogers* (Monterey, CA: Brooks/Cole, 1981), p. 30.

25 Daniel Goleman, "Positive Denial: The Case for Not Facing Reality" (Richard S. Lazarus interviewed by Daniel Goleman), *Psychology Today* (November 1979), p. 45.

26 Ibid., p. 60.

27 Wolpe, *Our Useless Fears*, p. 50.

28 A. Caponigro, "The Miracle of the Breath," *Body, Mind, and Spirit* (May 1996), p. 35.

29 Linehan, *Skills Training Manual*, pp. 170–171.

30 Herbert Benson, *The Relaxation Response* (New York: William Morrow, 1976), p. 78.

31 Stacy Taylor, *Living Well with a Hidden Disability* (Oakland, CA: New Harbinger Publications, 1999), p. 189.

32 Michael J. Norden, *Beyond Prozac* (New York: HarperCollins, 1995), p. 75.

33 George Leonard and Michael Murphy, *The Life We Are Given, Long Term Program for Realizing the Potential of Body, Mind, Heart, and Soul* (New York: G.P. Putnam, 1995), p. 118.

34 Susan Jeffers, *Feel the Fear and Do It Anyway* (New York: Fawcett Columbine, 1987), pp. 33–46.

35 Ibid., pp. 4–5.

36 Ibid., pp. 21–30.

37 Romweber, *Understanding the Emotional Experience*.

38 Louden, *The Woman's Comfort Book*, p. 28.

39 Linehan, *Skills Training Manual*, pp. 92–93.

40 Marsha Linehan, *Cognitive-Behavioral Treatment of Borderline Personality Disorder* (New York: Guilford Press, 1993), p. 150.

41 Ibid.

42 Edward Hallowell, *Connect* (New York: Pantheon, 1999).

43 Salvatore Maddi and Suzanne Kobasa, *The Hardy Executive: Health under Stress* (Homewood, IL: Dow Jones-Irwin, 1984), pp. 27–28.

44 Romweber, *Understanding the Emotional Experience.*

45 Judith McKay and Nancee Hirano, *The Chemotherapy and Radiation Therapy Survival Guide* (Oakland, CA: New Harbinger, 1998), p. 116.

46 Nancy Etcoff, *Survival of the Prettiest* (New York: Doubleday, 1999), p. 124.

47 Linehan, *Cognitive Behavioral Treatment*, p. 150.

48 Romweber, *Understanding the Emotional Experience.*

49 Ibid.

50 Louden, *The Woman's Comfort Book*, p. 2.

51 Linehan, *Cognitive Behavioral Treatment*, p. 148.

52 Linehan, *Skills Training Manual*, p. 96.

53 Leonard and Murphy, *The Life We Are Given*, p. 191.

54 Linehan, *Skills Training Manual*, p. 98.

55 Leonard and Murphy, *The Life We Are Given*, p. 194.

56 Taylor, *Living Well*, p. 185.

57 Romweber, *Understanding the Emotional Experience.*

58 Ibid.

59 M. Scott Peck, *The Road Less Traveled* (New York: Phoenix Press, Walker and Co., 1978), p. 43.

60 Taylor, *Living Well*, p. 186.

Chapter Eight — The Last Tangle

1 Shelley Taylor, "Adjustment to Threatening Events," *American Psychologist*, November 1983, 1161–1173.

2 Elizabeth Gilbert, "Losing Is Not an Option," *Reader's Digest*, March 2000, pp. 100–106.

3 Roxane L. Silver and Camille B. Wortman, "Coping with Undesirable Life Events," in *Human Helplessness, Theory and Applications*, ed. Judy Garber and Martin Seligman (New York: Academic Press, Inc., 1980), p. 317.

4 Philip Zimbardo and Floyd Ruch, *Psychology and Life* (Glenview, Illinois: Scott, Foresman and Company, 1977), p. 566.

5 Taylor, "Adjustment to Threatening Events," p. 1163; Victor Frankl, *Man's Search for Meaning* (New York: Washington Square Press, 1963).

6 Taylor, "Adjustment to Threatening Events," p. 1163.

7 Alan Monat, James Averill, and Richard Lazarus, "Anticipatory Stress and Coping Reactions Under Various Conditions of Uncertainty," *Journal of Personality and Social Psychology*, 1971, 24:237–253.

8 Richard S. Lazarus, *Psychological Stress and the Coping Process* (New York: McGraw-Hill Book Company, 1966), p. 187.

9 Judith McKay and Nancee Hirano, *The Chemotherapy & Radiation Therapy Survival Guide* (Oakland, CA: New Harbinger Publications, Inc., 1998), p. 116.

10 Sadick and Richardson, *Your Hair, Helping to Keep It*, pp. 61–62.

11 Ibid., p. 170.

12 Ibid., p. 112.
13 David Drum, *Making the Chemotherapy Decision* (Chicago: Contemporary Books, 1996), p. 151.
14 Sadick and Richardson, *Your Hair*, p. 173.
15 Corson, *Fashions in Hair*, p. 581.
16 Cooper, *Hair, Sex, Society, Symbolism*, pp. 53–56.
17 Renata Polt, "Hair Apparent," in *American Health*, June, 1994, p. 18.
18 Jojuan J. Lamorreaia, "Great Comebacks," *Essence* (April l993), 75–76.
19 Delma Heyn, "Are You Your Hair?" *Self*, February l997, p.128.
20 Ibid., p.129.
21 Romweber, *The Emotional Experience of Hair Loss.*
22 R. Freedman, *Beauty Bound* (Lexington, MA: D. C. Heath and Company, 1986), p. 74.
23 Ibid., pp. 28–29.
24 Sadick and Richardson, *Your Hair*, p. 3.
25 T. Cash, "Losing Hair, Losing Points? The Effects of Male Pattern Baldness on Social Impression Formation," *Journal of Applied Social Psychology*, 1990, 20: 154–167.
26 Victor Frankl, *The Doctor and the Soul* (New York: Alfred A. Knopf, 1965), pp.107–109.
27 Ibid., pp. 107–108.
28 Taylor, "Adjustment to Threatening Events," p. 1171.

Chapter Nine — Myth, Magic, and Medicine

1 Cyril P. Bryan (trans.), *The Papyrus Ebers* (London: Geoffrey Bles, 1930), p. 151.
2 Ibid., pp. 152–153.
3 Ibid., p. 156.
4 Alexander Rowland, *The Human Hair* (London: Piper Brothers, 1853), pp. 67–68.
5 Ibid., p. 68.
6 Ibid., p. 69–70.
7 C. Henri Leonard, *The Hair, Its Growth, Care, Diseases and Treatment* (Detroit: George S. Davis, 1881), pp. 147–149.
8 Ibid., p. 148.
9 Ibid., p. 149.
10 Ibid., p. 152.
11 Oscar L. Levin and Howard T. Behrman, *Your Hair and Its Care* (New York: Emerson Books, 1947), p. 74.
12 Ibid., p. 99, pp. 155 –164.
13 Ibid., p. 80.
14 Ibid., pp. 85–98.
15 Ibid., p. 92.
16 Ibid., pp. 97-98.
17 Ibid., p. 102.

18 Ibid., pp. 144–150.

19 Rodney Dawber and Dominique Van Neste, *Hair and Scalp Disorders* (Philadelphia: J.B. Lippincott Company, 1995), p. 25; Maria K. Hordinsky, *Hair Loss in Women* [video] (Secaucus, NJ: Network for Continuing Medical Education, 1995).

20 Dawber and Van Neste, *Hair and Scalp Disorders*, pp. 16–17.

21 Ibid., p. 248.

22 Sadick and Richardson, *Your Hair, Helping to Keep It*, pp. 40–42.

23 G. C. Lyketsos, J. Stratigos, G. Tawil, M. Psaras, C. G. Lyketsos, "Hostile Personality Characteristics, Dysthymic States and Neurotic Symptoms in Urticaria, Psoriasis and Alopecia," *Psychotherapy Psychosomatics*, 1985, 44:122–131.

24 A. Jarrett, E. Johnson, and R. Spearman, "Abnormal Hair Growth in Man," in *The Physiology and Pathophysiology of the Skin*, ed. A. Jarrett (New York: Academic Press, 1977), pp. 1530–1532.

25 Hordinsky. *Hair Loss.*

26 Jarrett, Johnson, and Spearman, *Abnormal Hair Growth*, p. 1525.

27 U. Schumacher-Stock, "Estrogen Treatment of Hair Diseases," in *Hair Research*, eds. C. Orfanos, W. Montagna, and G. Stuttgen (New York: Springer-Verlag, 1979), p. 318.

28 H. Baden, *Diseases of the Hair and Nails* (Chicago: Year Book Medical Publishers, 1987), p. 123.

29 Ibid., p. 129.

30 Sadick and Richardson, *Your Hair*, p. 18.

31 Dawber and Van Neste, *Hair and Scalp Disorders*, p. 106.

32 Ibid., p. 88.

33 Baden, *Diseases of the Hair*, pp. 161–164; Sadick and Richardson, *Your Hair*, p. 40.

34 Ibid., pp. 40–42.

35 Dawber and Van Neste, *Hair and Scalp Disorders*, p. 16.

36 Jeanine Barone, "Coping With Hair Loss," *Better Homes and Gardens*, September 1997, p.104.

37 Hordinsky. *Hair Loss.*

38 Kenneth A. Buchwach and Raymond J. Konior, *Contemporary Hair Transplant Surgery* (New York: Thieme Medical Publishers, Inc., 1997), p. 8.

39 Toby G. Mayer and Richard W. Fleming, *Aesthetic and Reconstructive Surgery of the Scalp* (Baltimore: Mosby Year Book, 1992), pp. 75–91.

40 James M. Swinehart, *Color Atlas of Hair Restoration Surgery* (Stamford, CT: Appleton and Lange, 1996), p. 93; Mayer and Fleming, *Aesthetic and Reconstructive Surgery*, pp. 215–239.

41 Swinehart, *Color Atlas*, p. 109.

42 Ibid., p. 193; Mayer and Fleming, *Aesthetic and Reconstructive Surgery*, pp. 93–213.

43 Sadick and Richardson, *Your Hair*, p. 132.

44 Mayer and Fleming, *Aesthetic and Reconstructive Surgery*, pp. 75–91.

45 Walter P. Unger, *Hair Transplantation* (New York: Marcel Dekker, 1980), p. 6.

46 Ibid., p. 27.
47 Buchwach & Konior, *Contemporary Hair*, pp. 151-167; Sadick and Richardson, Your Hair, pp. 126–128.
48 Swinehart, *Hair Restoration Surgery*, p. 93-107.
49 Sadick and Richardson, *Your Hair*, p. 130.
50 Mayer and Fleming, *Aesthetic and Reconstructive Surgery*, pp. 215–217.
51 Sadick and Richardson, *Your Hair*, p. 129.
52 Mayer and Fleming, *Aesthetic and Reconstructive Surgery*, p. 218.
53 Swinehart, *Hair Restoration Surgery*, p. 99.
54 Sadick and Richardson, Y*our Hair*, p. 131.
55 Ibid., Swinehart, *Hair Restoration Surgery*, pp. 97–99.
56 Swinehart, *Hair Restoration Surgery*, p. 99.
57 Sadick and Richardson, *Your Hair*, p. 131.
58 Swinehart, *Hair Restoration Surgery*, pp. 109–122.
59 Ibid., p. 113.
60 Ibid., pp. 225–226
61 Ibid., p. 193.
62 Sadick and Richardson, *Your Hair*, p. 132.
63 Mayer and Fleming, *Aesthetic and Reconstructive Surgery*, pp. 93–203.
64 Ibid., pp. 193-212; Walter P. Unger, "Surgical Approaches to Hair Loss," in *Disorders of Hair Growth, Diagnosis and Treatment*, ed. Elise A. Olsen (New York: McGraw-Hill, Inc., 1994), pp. 372–373.
65 Sadick and Richardson, *Your Hair*, p. 132.
66 Unger, *Hair Transplantation*, pp. 151–152
67 Sadick and Richardson, *Your Hair*, p. 134.
68 Ibid., pp. 138–139.
69 Ibid., p. 139.
70 Swinehart, *Hair Restoration Surgery*, pp. 373–375.
71 Unger, "Surgical Approaches to Hair Loss," p. 373.
72 Buchwach and Konior, *Contemporary Hair*, p. 8.
73 Sadick and Richardson, *Your Hair*, p. 119.
74 Maria K. Hordinsky, "Alopecia areata," in *Disorders of Hair Growth*, ed. Elise A. Olsen (New York: McGraw-Hill, 1994) pp. 206–207.
75 Ibid.
76 Dawber and Van Neste, *Hair and Scalp Disorders*, pp. 187–188
77 Hordinsky, *Hair Loss.*
78 Dawber and Van Neste, *Hair and Scalp Disorders*, p. 105.
79 Ibid.
80 Ibid.
81 Karen L. Wagner, "Get to the Root of Hair Disorders," *Dermatology Insights*, Spring 2000, pp. 27–28.
82 Pat Beach, "Spraying for Deliverance," *Gentlemen's Quarterly*, January 1998, pp. 80–82.
83 Ron Geraci, "A Little More on the Top," *Men's Health*, September 1998, pp. 130–135.
84 Beach, "Spraying for Deliverance," p. 80.
85 Dawber and Van Neste, *Hair and Scalp Disorders*, p. 187.

86   Ibid., p. 189
87   Hordinsky, "Alopecia areata," p. 206.
88   Ibid.
89   Wagner, "Get to the Root of Hair Disorders," pp. 27–28.
90   Geraci, "A Little More on Top," pp. 130–135.
91   Hordinsky, "Alopecia areata," p. 276.
92   Ibid.; Sadick and Richardson, *Your Hair*, p. 102.
93   Hordinsky, "Alopecia areata," p. 276.
94   Ibid., pp. 207-208.
95   Geraci, "A Little More on Top," p. 135.
96   John Sedgwick, "Roots," *Gentlemen's Quarterly*, May 1999, p. 218.
97   Ibid., p. 216.
98   Ibid., p. 239.
99   "Making Old Follicles Young Again," *Newsweek*, December 7, 1998, p. 60.

Chapter Ten — Hair Peace

1   Romweber, *Understanding the Emotional Experience of Hair Loss.*
2   Ibid.
3   Ibid.
4   Judi Johnson and Linda Klein, *I Can Cope: Staying Healthy with Cancer* (Minneapolis, MN: Chronimed Publishing, 1994), p. 125.
5   Binder, *Muffs and Morals*, pp. 105–106.
6   Cooper, *Hair: Sex, Society, Symbolism*, p. 121.
7   Sadick and Richardson, *Your Hair*, p. 136.
8   Jonathan Zizmor and John Foreman, *Super Hair, The Doctor's Book of Beautiful Hair* (New York: Berkley Publishing Corporation, 1978), pp. 156–157.
9   Sadick and Richardson, *Your Hair*, p. 136.
10   Ibid.
11. Cooper, *Hair*, p. 168.
12   Zizmor and Foreman, *Super Hair*, p. 157.
13   *Beauty Trends: Fashion Hair for Every Woman, Every Style* [wig catalogue]; P.O. Box 9323; Hialeah, Florida 33013-9323.
14   Zizmor and Foreman, *Super Hair*, p. 157.
15   Ibid., pp. 157–158.
16   Sadick and Richardson, *Your Hair*, pp. 136–137.
17   Zizmor and Foreman, *Super Hair*, p. 158.
18   Sadick and Richardson, *Your Hair*, p. 137.
19   Zizmor and Foreman, *Super Hair*, p. 158.
20   Ibid.
21   Corson, *Fashions in Hair*, pp. 632–633.
22   Gale Hansen, "Beauty 411: Fake Out" in *Harper's Bazaar*, March 1999, p. 250.
23. Romweber, *Understanding the Emotional Experience of Hair Loss.*
24. Sadick and Richardson, *Your Hair*, pp. 137–138; Hansen, "Beauty 411," p. 250.

25 Ibid., p. 138.
26 Hansen, "Beauty 411," p. 250.
27 Ibid., p. 252.
28 Ibid.
29 Corson, *Fashions in Hair*, p. 601.
30 Tamala Edwards, "Hair Down to There" in *Time Magazine*, 2 February 1999, p. 73.
31 Zizmor and Foreman, *Super Hair*, p. 157.
32 Corson, Fashions in *Hair*, pp. 277–278.
33 Ibid., p. 581.
34 Mike Michaelson, "How Your Man Can Crown Himself With Glory . . . When His Hairline Starts Retreating," in *Today's Health*, March 1973, p. 19.
35 Joe Kita, "Who Wants to Join the Hair Club for Men" (edited by Ron Geraci) in *Men's Health*, June 1999, p. 115.
36 Ibid.
37 Sadick and Richardson, *Your Hair*, p. 137.
38 Amy Spindler, "The Beauty Diagnosis" in *Vogue*, April 1999, pp. 271–274.
39 Ibid., p. 271.
40 Ibid., p. 274.
41 Polt, "Hair Apparent," pp. 18–23.
42 Ibid., p.23.
43 Stephen Franzoi, Joan Anderson, and Stephen Frommelt, "Individual Differences in Men's Perceptions of and Reactions to Thinning Hair," *Journal of Social Psychology*, 1990, 130(2), 209–218.
44 Romweber, *Understanding the Emotional Experience of Hair Loss*.

REFERENCES

Ackerman, Diane (1994). *A Natural History of Love*. New York: Random House.

Aldrich, Maria (1993). *Hair*. In Joseph Epstein (Ed.), The Best American Essays 1993. New York: Ticknor and Fields, pp. 1–7.

Allione, Tsultrim (1984). *Women of Wisdom*. London: Routledge & Kegan Paul.

Al-Mutanabbi (1967). Verses composed in the poet's youth. In A. J. Arberry (trans.) *Poems of Al-Mutanabbi*. Great Britain: Cambridge University Press.

Andresen, J. (1980). Rapunzel: The symbolism of the cutting of hair. *Journal of the American Psychoanalytic Association*, 28(1), 68–88.

Baden, H. (1987). *Diseases of the Hair and Nails*. Chicago: Year Book Medical Publishers.

Baron, Robert, and Byrne, Donn (1981). *Social Psychology: Understanding Human Interaction*. Boston: Allyn and Bacon, Inc.

Barone, Jeanine (1997, September). Coping with hair loss. *Better Homes and Gardens*, p. 104.

Beach, Pat (1998, January). Spraying for deliverance. *Gentlemen's Quarterly*, pp. 80–82.

Benson, Herbert (1976). *The Relaxation Response*. New York: William Morrow and Co.

Berg, C. (1951). The unconscious significance of hair. *The International Journal of Psychoanalysis*, 17, 73–88.

Bernstein, Marcel (1976). *The Nuns*. Philadelphia: J. B. Lippincott.

Beswick, D. (1997). *Bald Men Always Come Out on Top*. St. Augustine, FL: Ama Publishing.

Binder, Pearl (1954). *Muffs and Morals*. New York: William Morrow & Company.

Bohannon, P. (1938). Edward B. Tylor: *Researches into the Early History of Mankind*. Chicago: The University of Chicago Press.

Bridges, William (1980). *Transitions: Making Sense of Life's Changes*. Reading, MA: Addison-Wesley Publishing Company.

Boynton, Henry W. (1931). *The Complete Poetical Works of Pope*. New York: Houghton Mifflin Company.

Brislin, R. W., and Lewis, S. A. (1968). Dating and physical attractiveness:

replication. *Psychological Reports*, 22, 976.

Brooks, Geraldine (1995). *Nine Parts of Desire: The Hidden World of Islamic Women*. New York: Doubleday.

Bryan, Cyril P. (trans) (1930). *The Papyrus Ebers*. London: Geoffrey Bles.

Buchwald, Kenneth A., and Konior R. J. (1997). *Contemporary Hair Transplant Surgery*. New York: Thieme Medical Publishers, Inc.

Byron, Lord (1928). Maid of Athens, ere we part. *Romantic Poetry of the Early Nineteenth Century*. New York: Charles Scribner's Sons.

Caligor, L., and May, R. (1968). *Dreams and Symbols: Man's Unconscious Language*. New York: Basic Books.

Campbell, B. G. (1966). *Human Evolution: An Introduction to Man's Adaptations*. Chicago: Aldine Publishing Company.

Campbell-Jones, Susan (1979). *In Habit: An Anthropological Study of Working Nuns*. London: Faber & Faber.

Caponigro, Andy (1996, May). The miracle of the breath. *Body, Mind, and Spirit*, pp. 35–38.

Cash, Tom (1990). Losing hair, losing points? The effects of male pattern baldness on social impression formation. *Journal of Applied Social Psychology*, 20, 154–167.

Chapman, Penny, and Masters, Sue (Executive Producers), and Ken Cameron (Director) (1991). *Brides of Christ* [Film]. Santa Sabina College, Sydney, New Southy Wales, Australia. Australian Broadcasting Corporation and Roadshow Coate and Carroll.

Conway, Moncure (1879). *Demonology and Devil-Lore*. London: Ballantyne Press.

Cooper, Wendy (1971). *Hair: Sex, Society, Symbolism*. New York: Stein and Day.

Corbin, A. (1982). *Le Miasme et la Jonquille* [The Foul and the Fragrant]. Paris, France: Aubier Montaigne.

Corson, Richard (1965). *Fashions in Hair*. London: Peter Owen Limited.

Cousins, Norman (1979). *Anatomy of an Illness as Perceived by the Patient*. New York: W.W. Norton and Company.

Craig, C. (1953). The first epistle to the Corinthians. In G. Buttrick, W. Bowie, J. Knox, N. Harmon, P. Sherer, S. Terrien (Eds), *The Interpreter's Bible*. New York: Abingdon-Cokesbury Press.

Crawley, E. (1927). *The Mystic Rose*, vol. 1. London: Boni and Liveright.

Crooke, W. (1896). *Folklore of Northern India*. Nai Sarak, Delhi: Munshiram Manoharlal.

Cunnington, C. Willette (1973). *Feminine Attitudes in the Nineteenth Century*. New York: Haskell House Publishers Ltd.

Darwin, Charles (1871). *The Descent of Man and Selection in Relation to Sex*. New York: Modern Library.

Darwin, Charles (1936). *The Origin of the Species and the Descent of Man*. New York: The Modern Library.

Dawber, R., and Van Neste, D. (1995). *Hair and Scalp Disorders*. Philadelphia: J. B. Lippincott Company.

Dawood, N. J. (trans) (1974). *Koran* (24:30). New York: Penguin Books.

Derrett, J. D. (1973). Religious hair. *Man* (N.S.), 8, 100–103.

Douglas, M. (1970). *Natural Symbols*. London: The Cresset Press.

Drum, David (1996). *Making the Chemotherapy Decision*. Chicago: Contemporary Books.

Dunn-Mascetti, Manuela (1994). *Saints, The Chosen Few*. New York: Ballantine Books.

Eder, M. D. (1925). A note on shingling. *International Journal of Psychoanalysis*, 6, 325–326.

Edwards, Tamala (1999, February 2). *Time Magazine*, p. 73.

Ellis, Albert (1997). *How to Control Your Anger Before It Controls You*. Sebaucus, NJ: Carol Publishing Group.

Etcoff, Nancy (1999). Survival of the Prettiest. New York: Doubleday.

Ellis, H. (1938). *Psychology of Sex: A Manual for Students*. New York: Emerson Books.

Faraone, C. A. (1992). *Talisman and Trojan Horses*. New York: Oxford University Press.

Fenigstein, Allan (1979). Self-consciousness, self-attention, and social interaction. *Journal of Personality and Social Psychology*, 37, 75–86.

Festinger, L. (1954). A theory of social comparison processes. *Human Relations*, 7, 117–140.

Field, S. and McCormick, K. (Producers), and Schumacher, J. (Director) (1991). *Dying Young* [Film]. Hollywood, CA: 20th Century Fox.

Finck, Henry. (1912). *Romantic Love and Personal Beauty*. New York: The Macmillan Company.

Firth, R. (1973). *Symbols, Public and Private*. Ithaca, NY: Cornell University Press.

Fisher, H. (1992). *Anatomy of Love*. New York: W. W. Norton and Company.

Frankl, V. (1965). *The Doctor and the Soul*. New York: Alfred A. Knopf.

Franzoi, S., Anderson, J., and Frommelt, S. (1990). Individual differences in man's perceptions of and reactions to thinning hair. *Journal of Social Psychology*, 130(2), 209–218.

Frazier, J. G. (1940). *The Golden Bough, a Study in Magic and Religion*, Vol. 2. New York: Macmillan & Co.

Freedman, R. (1986). *Beauty Bound*. Lexington, MA: D. C. Heath and Company

Gastor, T. H. (1955). *The Holy and the Profane*. New York: William Sloane Associates.

Genesis (24:65) in *The Torah, The First Five Books of Moses* (1962). Philadelphia: The Jewish Publication Society of America

Geraci, Ron (1998, September). A little more on top. *Men's Health*, pp. 130–135.

Gilbert, Elizabeth (2000, March). Losing is not an option. *Reader's Digest*, pp. 100–106.

Goleman, Daniel (1979, November). Positive denial: The case for not facing reality. (Richard S. Lazarus interviewed by Daniel Goleman). *Psychology Today*, pp. 45–60.

Goodhart, C. B. (1960). The evolutionary significance of human hair patterns and skin coloring. *Advancement of Science*, 17, 53–59.

Goodwin, Jan (1994). *Price of Honor, Muslim Women Lift the Veil of Silence on the Islamic World*. Boston, MA: Little, Brown and Company.

Gregor, A. S. (1972). *Witchcraft and Magic*. New York: Charles Scribner's Sons.

Grimm, J., and Grimm, W. (1944). *Rapunzel. The Complete Grimm's Fairy Tales*. New York: Pantheon Books.

Gundry, Patricia. (1988). *Woman be Free*. Grand Rapids, MI: Zondervan Publishing House.

Hallowell, Edward M. (1999). *Connect*. New York: Pantheon Books.

Hallpike, C. R. (1969). Social hair. *Man*, 4, 256–264.

Hansen, Gale (1999, March). Beauty 411: Fake out. *Harper's Bazaar*, p. 250.

Hatfield, E., and Sprecher, S. (1986). *Mirror, Mirror . . . The Importance of Looks in Everyday Life*. Albany: State University of New York Press.

Hayes, B. (Executive Producer) and Wilcher, D. (Producer), and Streb, K. (Director and Writer) (1999). *The Bald Truth* [Film]. Commerce, CA: Discovery Channel Video.

Hershman, P. (1974). Hair, sex and dirt. *Man*, (N.S.), 9, 275–298.

Heyn, Dalma (1997, February). Are you your hair? *Self*, pp. 128–131.

Hordinsky, Maria (1994). Alopecia areata. In E. Olsen (Ed.), *Disorders of Hair Growth, Diagnosis and Treatment*. New York: McGraw-Hill.

Hordinsky, Maria (1995). *Hair Loss in Women* [video]. Secaucus, NJ: Network for Continuing Medical Education.

Hurley, James B. (1981). *Man and Woman in Biblical Perspective*. Grand Rapids, Michigan: Zondervan Publishing House.

Jampolsky, Gerald, and Cirincione, Diane (1993). *Change Your Mind, Change Your Life*. New York, NY: Bantam Books.

Jarrett, A., Johnson, E., and Spearman, R. (1977). Abnormal hair growth in man. In A. Jarrett (Ed.), *The Physiology and Pathophysiology of the Skin*. New York: Academic Press.

Jeffers, Susan (1987). *Feel the Fear and Do It Anyway*. New York: Fawcett Columbine.

Johnson, J., and Klein, L (1994). *I Can Cope*. Minneapolis, MN: Chronimed Publishing.

Jolley, W. (1999). *A Setback is a Setup for a Comeback*. New York, NY: St. Martin's Press.

Kita, Joe (edited by Ron Geraci) (1999, June). Who wants to join the Hair Club for Men? *Men's Health*, p. 115.

Kittredge, G. L. (1929). *Witchcraft in Old New England*. Cambridge, MA: Harvard University Press.

Lamorreaia, J. (1993, April). Great comebacks. *Essence*, pp. 75–76.

Laver, J. (1945). *Taste and Fashion*. London: George G. Harrap and Company Ltd.

Lazarus, Richard (1966). *Psychological Stress and the Coping Process*. New York: McGraw-Hill Book Company.

Leach, E. R. (1957). Magical hair. *Journal of the Royal Anthropological Institute*, 88 (Part 2), 147–164.

Lennon, John, and McCartney, Paul (Composers) (1966). Here, There, and Everywhere [song]. Mayfair, London: Northern Songs Limited.

Leonard, C. Henri (1881). *The Hair, its Growth, Care, Diseases and Treatment*. Detroit: George S. Davis.

Leonard, George, and Murphy, Michael (1995). *The Life We Are Given, A Long Term Program for Realizing the Potential of Body, Mind, Heart, and Soul*. New York: G.P. Putnams's Sons.

Levin, O., and Behrman, H. (1947). *Your Hair and its Care*. New York: Emerson Books.

Linehan, Marsha (1993). *Cognitive Behavioral Treatment of Borderline Personality Disorder*. New York: The Guilford Press.

Linehan, Marsha (1993). *Skills Training Manual for Treating Borderline Personality Disorder*. New York: The Guilford Press.

Louden, Jennifer (1992). *The Women's Comfort Book*. San Francisco, CA: Harper.

Lyketsos, G. C., Stratigos, J., Tawil, G., Psaras, M., Lyketsos, C. G. (1985). Hostile personality characteristics, dysthymic states and neurotic symptoms in urticaria, psoriasis and alopecia. *Psychotherapy Psychosomatics*, 44, 122–131.

Lynden, Patricia (interviewing Loretta LaRoche) (2001, March/April). Queen of the stress busters. *New Age*, p. 74.

Maddi, Salvatore, and Kobasa, Suzanne (1984). *The Hardy Executive: Health Under Stress*. Homewood, Illinois: Dow Jones-Irwin.

Mayer, T. G., and Fleming, R. W. (1992). *Aesthetic and Reconstructive Surgery of the Scalp*. Baltimore: Mosby Year Book.

McKay, Judith, and Hirano, Nancee (1998). *The Chemotherapy & Radiation Therapy Survival Guide*. Oakland, CA: New Harbinger Publications, Inc.

Michaelson, Mike (1973, March). How your man can crown himself with glory . . . when his hairline starts retreating. *Today's Health*, pp. 16–19+.

Miller, J. (1978). *The Healing Power of Grief.* New York: The Seabury Press.

Miller, Suzanne (1980). Why having control reduces stress: If I can stop the roller coaster, I don't want to get off. In J. Garber and M. Seligman (Eds.), *Human Helplessness, Theory and Applications.* New York: Academic Press.

Miller, Timothy (1991). *The Hippies and American Values.* Knoxville: The University of Tennessee Press.

Min, J., Stratte-McClure, J., Nolan, C., Biddle, N. and Vlahou, T. (1996, September 30). Trouble in Monaco. *People*, pp. 71–76.

Minai, N. (1981). *Women in Islam: Tradition and Transition in the Middle East.* New York: Seaview Books.

Monat, A., Averill, J., and Lazarus, R. (1971). Anticipatory stress and coping reactions under various conditions of uncertainty. *Journal of Personality and Social Psychology*, 24, 237–253.

Montagna, W. (1965). The skin. *Scientific America*, 212, 53–59.

Morris, Desmond (1967). *The Naked Ape.* London: Jonathan Cape.

Murphy, Cullen (1998). *The World According to Eve.* New York: Houghton Mifflin Company.

Noles, S., Cash, T. F., and Winstead, B. A. (1985). Body image, physical attractiveness, and depression. *Journal of Consulting and Clinical Psychology*, 53(1), 88–94.

Norden, Michael (1995). *Beyond Prozac.* New York: HarperCollins Publishers.

Nye, Robert D. (1981). *Three Psychologies: Perspectives from Freud, Skinner, and Rogers.* Monterey, CA: Brooks/Cole Publishing Company.

Peck, M. Scott (1984). *The Road Less Traveled.* New York: Phoenix Press, Walker and Company.

Pines, Maya (1980). "Psychological hardiness: The role of challenge in health." *Psychology Today*, pp. 34–44, 98.

Poiret, Paul (1967). Individuality in dress, the secret of the well-dressed woman. In Jane Trahey (Ed.), *Harper's Bazaar.* New York: Random House.

Polt, Renata (1994, June). Hair apparent. *American Health*, pp. 18–23.

Qur'an (Surah, XXXIII:53), trans. by M. H. Shakir (1993). Elmhurst, NY: Tahrike Tarsile Qur'an, Inc.

Rich, M., and Cash, T. (1993). The American image of beauty: Media representations of hair color for four decades. *Sex Roles*, 29, Nos. 1/2, pp. 113–124.

Romweber, S. (1996). *Understanding the Emotional Experience of Scalp Hair Loss.* Ph.D. dissertation, Saybrook Graduate School and Research Center, San Francisco, CA.

Rowland, A. (1853). *The Human Hair.* London: Piper Brothers.

Ryback, T. (1993, November 15). Evidence of evil. *The New Yorker*, pp. 68–81.

Sadick, N., and Richardson, D. (1991). *Your Hair, Helping to Keep It.* Yonkers,

NY: Consumer Reports.

Sagay, Esi (1983). *African Hairstyles*. Portsmouth, New Hampshire: Heinemann.

Scanzoni, L., and Hardesty, N. (1986). *All We're Meant To Be*. Nashville, TN: Abington Press.

Schimmel, Selma, and Fox, Barry (1999). *Cancer Talk:Voices of Hope and Endurance*. New York: Broadway Books.

Schneider, S. (1984). *Jewish and Female*. New York: Simon and Schuster.

Schumacher-Stock, U. (1979). Estrogen treatment of hair diseases. In C. Orfanos, W. Montagna, and G. Stuttgen (Eds), *Hair Research*. New York: Springer-Verlag.

Sedgewick, John (1999, May). Roots. *Gentlemen's Quarterly*, pp. 214–219.

Sheier, Michael (1980). Effects of public and private self-consciousness on the public expression of personal beliefs. *Journal of Personality and Social Psychology*, 39(3), 514–521.

Silver, R., and Wortman, C. (1980). Coping with undesirable life events. In J. Garber and M. Seligman (Eds), *Human Helplessness, Theory and Applications*. New York: Academic Press.

Simos, B. (1979). *A Time to Grieve*. New York: Family Service Association of America.

Skeat, Walter W. (1965). *Malay Magic*. London: Frank Cass and Co. LTD.

Sourkes, B. (1982). "A Life of My Own," in *The Deepening Shade: Psychological Aspects of Life Threatening Illness*. Pittsburgh: University of Pittsburgh Press.

Spindler, Amy (1999, *Vogue*). The beauty diagnosis. *Vogue*, pp. 271–274.

Swinehart, James M. (1996). *Color Atlas of Hair Restoration Surgery*. Stamford, CT: Appleton and Lange.

Synnott, A. (1987). Shame and glory: A sociology of hair. *British Journal of Sociology*, 38(3), 381–413.

Tanner, Ira (1976). *The Gift of Grief*. New York: Hawthorne Books, Inc.

Taylor, Shelley (1983, November). Adjustment to threatening events. *American Psychologist*, pp. 1161–1173.

Taylor, Shelley (1989). Positive Illusions: *Creative Self-Deception and the Healthy Mind*. New York: Basic Books, Inc., Publishers.

Taylor, Stacy. (1999). *Living Well with a Hidden Disability*. Oakland, CA: New Harbinger Publications.

Tesser, A., and Brodie, M. (1971). A note on evaluation of a 'computer date.' *Psychonomic Science*, 23, 300.

"The First Epistle of Paul the Apostle to the Corinthians," *The Holy Bible* (Revised Standard Version). New York: Collins, 1973.

Toews, P. (1996). *Mennonites in American Society*, 1930–1970. Scottdale, Pennsylvania: Herald Press.

Trepp, Leo (1980). *The Complete Book of Jewish Observance*. New York: Behrman House, Inc./Summit Books.

Turk, Midge (1971). *The Buried Life*. New York: The World Publishing Company.

Unger, Walter P. (1980). *Hair Transplantation*. New York: Marcel Dekker.

Unger, Walter P. (1994). Surgical approaches to hair loss. In Elise A. Olsen (Ed.) *Disorders of Hair Growth, Diagnosis and Treatment*. New York: McGraw-Hill.

Wagner, Karen L. (2000, Spring). Get to the root of hair disorders. *Dermatology Insights*, pp. 27–28.

Walster, W., Aronson, V., Abrahams, D., and Rottman, L. (1966). Importance of physical attractiveness in dating behavior. *Journal of Personality and Social Psychology*, 4, 508–516.

Williamson, M. (1979). Powhatan hair. *Man*, 49(3), 392–419.

Wogalter, M., and Hosie, J. (1991). Effects of cranial and facial hair on perceptions of age and person. *The Journal of Social Psychology*, 131(4), 589–591.

Wolf, Naomi (1991). *The Beauty Myth*. New York: William Morrow and Company.

Wolpe, Joseph (with David Wolpe) (1981). *Our Useless Fears*. Boston: Houghton Mifflin Company.

Wong, Mary Gilligan (1983). *Nun, A Memoir of Mary Gilligan Wong*. San Diego: Harcourt Brace Jovanovich Publishers.

Yonge, Charlotte (1882). *Womankind*. New York: Macmillan and Company.

Zimbardo, P., and Ruch, F. (1977). P*sychology and Life*. Glenview, IL: Scott Foresman and Company.

Zizmor, Jonathan, and Foreman, John (1978). *Super Hair: The Doctor's Book of Beautiful Hair*. New York: Berkley Publishing Corporation.

INDEX

ABOUT THE AUTHOR

Sara Romweber has an A.A. in nursing from Manatee Community College, Bradenton, Florida, a B.S. in psychology from St. Joseph's College, North Windham, Maine, an M.Ed. in counseling from the University of North Carolina-Chapel Hill, and a Ph.D. in psychology from Saybrook Graduate School and Research Center (San Francisco).

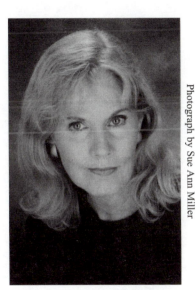

Photograph by Sue Ann Miller

She works as a psychotherapist in private practice in Chapel Hill, North Carolina, and a nurse-consultant at SAS Institute.

She maintains an active membership in the North Carolina Writer's Network.

Sara Romweber, Ph.D.

For a signed copy of this book, you may email Dr. Romweber at sromweber@intrex.net